T0173476

THE
HEDGEROW
APOTHECARY
FORAGER'S
HANDBOOK

THE HEDGEROW APOTHECARY FORAGER'S HANDBOOK

Copyright © Christine Iverson, 2022
Some text has been taken from *The Hedgerow Apothecary*

All rights reserved.

No part of this book may be reproduced by any means, nor transmitted, nor translated into a machine language, without the written permission of the publishers.

Christine Iverson has asserted her right to be identified as the author of this work in accordance with sections 77 and 78 of the Copyright, Designs and Patents Act 1988.

Condition of Sale
This book is sold subject to the condition that it shall not, by way of trade or otherwise, be lent, resold, hired out or otherwise circulated in any form of binding or cover other than that in which it is published and without a similar condition including this condition being imposed on the subsequent purchaser.

An Hachette UK Company
www.hachette.co.uk

Summersdale Publishers Ltd
Part of Octopus Publishing Group Limited
Carmelite House
50 Victoria Embankment
LONDON
EC4Y 0DZ
UK

www.summersdale.com

Printed and bound in China

ISBN: 978-1-80007-181-0

This FSC® label means that materials used for the product have been responsibly sourced

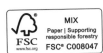

MIX
Paper | Supporting responsible forestry
FSC
www.fsc.org   FSC® C008047

Substantial discounts on bulk quantities of Summersdale books are available to corporations, professional associations and other organizations. For details contact general enquiries: telephone: +44 (0) 1243 771107 or email: enquiries@summersdale.com.

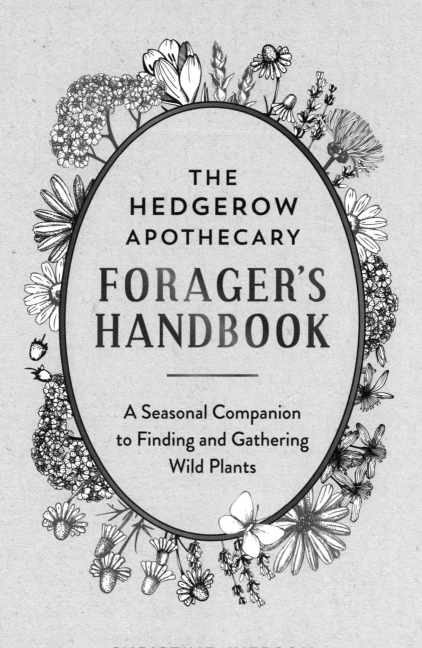

THE HEDGEROW APOTHECARY

FORAGER'S HANDBOOK

A Seasonal Companion
to Finding and Gathering
Wild Plants

CHRISTINE IVERSON

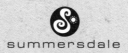

summersdale

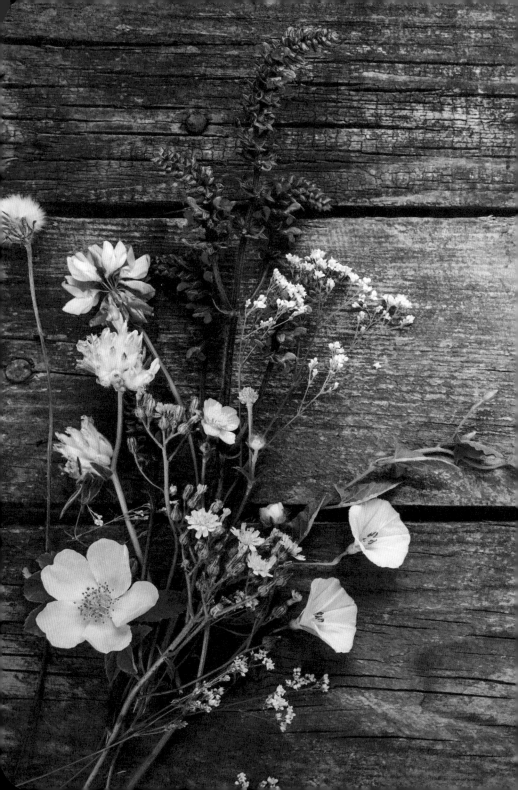

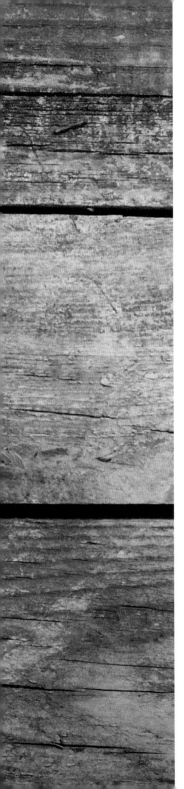

CONTENTS

7   About the Author

8   Introduction

10   Foraging Calendar

12   Foraging Toolkit

13   Foraging Etiquette

14   Kitchen Essentials

15   Conversions and Measurements

16   A Brief History of "Cunning Folk"

18   January, February, March

40   April, May, June

76   July, August, September

126   October, November, December

148   Festivals

155   Final Thoughts

156   Index

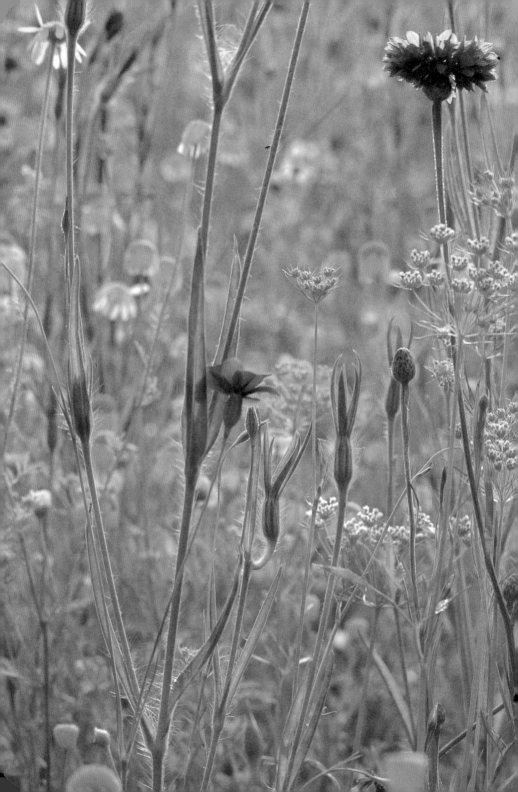

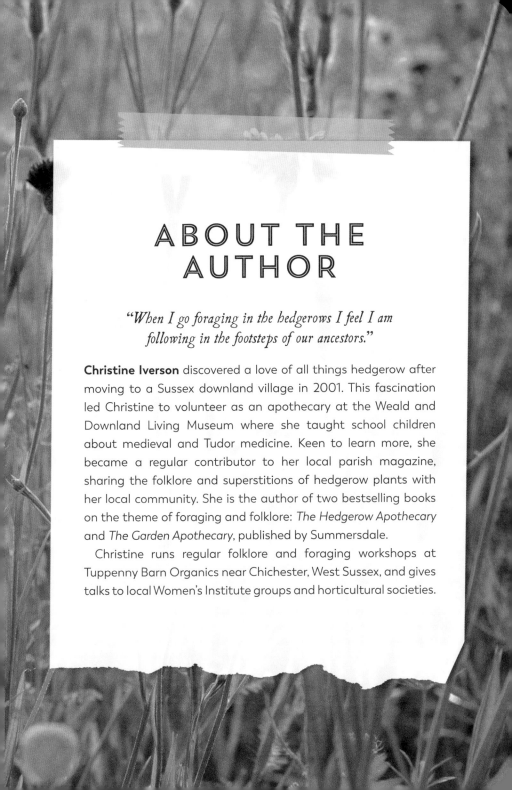

ABOUT THE AUTHOR

*"When I go foraging in the hedgerows I feel I am
following in the footsteps of our ancestors."*

Christine Iverson discovered a love of all things hedgerow after
moving to a Sussex downland village in 2001. This fascination
led Christine to volunteer as an apothecary at the Weald and
Downland Living Museum where she taught school children
about medieval and Tudor medicine. Keen to learn more, she
became a regular contributor to her local parish magazine,
sharing the folklore and superstitions of hedgerow plants with
her local community. She is the author of two bestselling books
on the theme of foraging and folklore: *The Hedgerow Apothecary*
and *The Garden Apothecary*, published by Summersdale.

Christine runs regular folklore and foraging workshops at
Tuppenny Barn Organics near Chichester, West Sussex, and gives
talks to local Women's Institute groups and horticultural societies.

INTRODUCTION

People sometimes ask me, "Why go to the trouble of foraging when food and medicine is so readily available in supermarkets?"

Good question – why bother?

When you begin your foraging journey you'll discover that it is about so much more than identifying a few wild plants. It's about immersing yourself in the countryside, learning a skill that will probably take you many years to master and getting a taste for the social history that has shaped rural life. You'll find yourself becoming much more in tune with the seasons as you watch the progress of nature all around you. Not only is this great for your physical health, it's beneficial for your mental health as well. Foraging is an activity for the whole family – in fact, I would positively encourage you to teach your children the skills included in this book and they will hopefully pass them on to their own children. The added bonus is that you can gather some wild ingredients to make into simple remedies and recipes, which will give you immense satisfaction.

My foraging journey began when I moved to a small downland village in West Sussex. At this point my foraging knowledge was very limited, but the idea of food and medicine for free really fascinated me. Armed with a simple field guide, I cautiously ventured out into the hedgerows to see what I could find; needless to say I was soon hooked. That was over 20 years ago and I'm still foraging and learning!

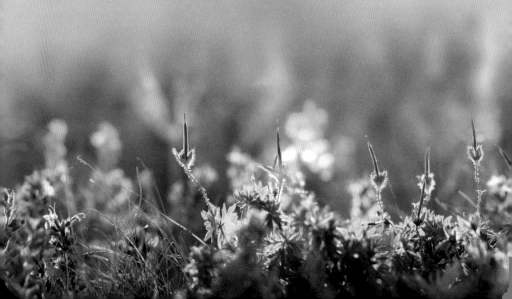

The Hedgerow Apothecary Forager's Handbook is the perfect companion on your foraging journey. It is helpfully arranged in seasons with clear photos to aid you with plant identification and handy pages for you to make notes or drawings of your own. It's a good idea to keep a note or a sketch of where you find something particularly interesting – every forager has a secret hedgerow where they can find the best sloes in preparation for that Christmas sloe gin (see page 132)!

Don't be afraid to dive in; start off with something easily identifiable such as blackberries to make into jam or vinegar. You'll soon feel confident to move on to something less familiar, and the more you look, the more you will find.

It is vital that you take personal responsibility for your safety when foraging. Many plants should not be used during pregnancy, on young children or babies, or on people with certain medical conditions. Consult your GP if you have any doubts. If you're not 100 per cent certain of what you're picking, don't pick it!

Be warned, though: once you start foraging, you'll never want to stop!

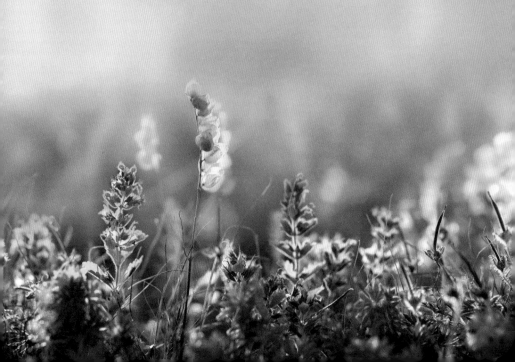

FORAGING CALENDAR

JANUARY, FEBRUARY, MARCH

Chickweed, common mallow leaves, common sorrel, cowberry, crow garlic, dandelion root, garlic mustard, ground elder, hairy bittercress, nettles, pignut, sheep's sorrel, silver birch sap, wild garlic, winter cress, wood sorrel

APRIL, MAY, JUNE

Beech leaves, borage, broom, chickweed, cleavers, common poppy, dandelion leaves and roots, dog rose flowers, elderflower, garlic mustard, ground elder, hawthorn blossom, hops, nettles, pignuts, sheep's sorrel, spearmint, sweet cicely, watercress, wild garlic, wild thyme, wood sorrel, yarrow

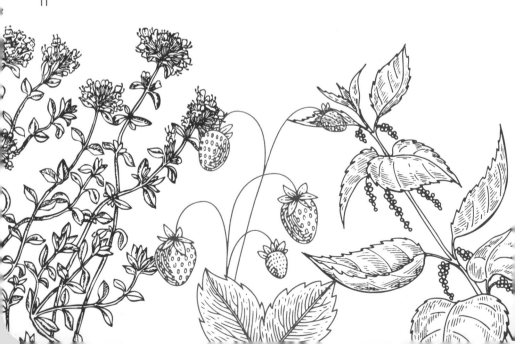

JULY, AUGUST, SEPTEMBER

Acorns, apples, beech nuts, bilberries, blackberries, burdock, camomile, chickweed, chicory, cleavers, common mallow, dandelion leaves and flowers, elderberry, fat hen, garlic mustard, gooseberries, hawthorn berries, hazelnuts, horseradish, juniper berries, nettle, plums, rowan berries, sheep's sorrel, spearmint, sweet chestnuts, sweet cicely, walnuts, wild cherries, wild strawberries, wild thyme, wood sorrel, yarrow

OCTOBER, NOVEMBER, DECEMBER

Chestnuts, chickweed, crab apples, hawthorn berries, horseradish, nettles, rosehips, sheep's sorrel, sloes, spearmint, sweet chestnuts, walnuts

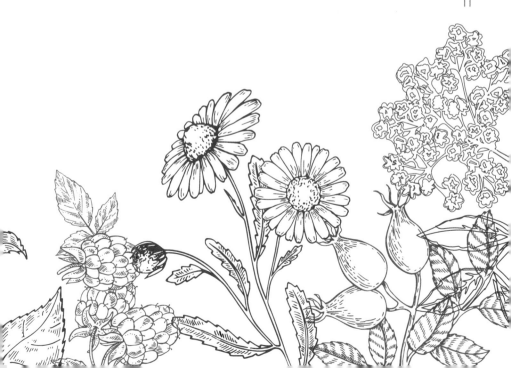

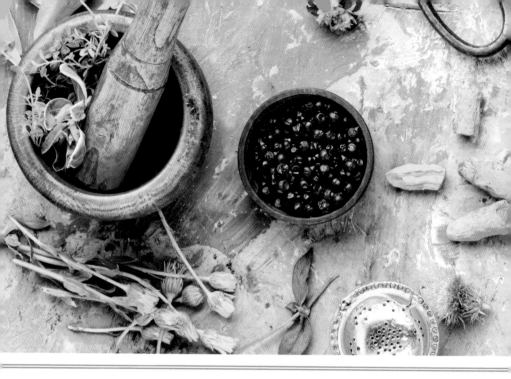

FORAGING TOOLKIT

- **A good pocket-sized field guide with clear pictures:** If you are not 100 per cent certain that you can correctly identify a plant, DO NOT PICK IT!

- **Clothing:** You will inevitably encounter nettles and brambles, so long trousers, long sleeves, gardening gloves and sturdy boots are recommended.

- **Secateurs or scissors:** These are useful for collecting samples and cause less damage to the plants. I wouldn't advise carrying a knife for safety's sake.

- **Baskets:** These are best to transport soft fruit, keeping it in the best condition. And I always like to carry extra bags for those unexpected finds.

- **"Hooky stick":** My own invention – a long piece of garden cane with a large hook screwed into the end. This will gently pull the higher branches down to you, because the best fruits are always just out of reach! A walking cane will work just as well.

- **Pen or pencil:** So that you can make notes in your foraging handbook.

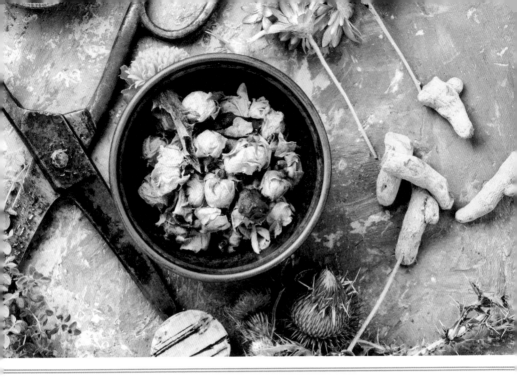

FORAGING ETIQUETTE

- **Location:** If you wish to forage on private land you MUST get permission from the landowner first. I find that the promise of some homemade goodies usually persuades them to welcome your visit. Avoid areas that have been contaminated by road pollution or fields that have been sprayed with pesticides or may have been contaminated by dogs.

- **Respect nature:** Pick no more than you need, leaving plenty for wildlife to enjoy. Try not to disturb habitats, and take all rubbish away with you. Stay away from any Sites of Special Scientific Interest (SSSIs) in the UK, as these are protected for a reason.

- **Do not pick endangered species:** (Your field guide should help you.) The digging up of roots is frowned upon unless they are abundant and a common species.

- **Be cautious when trying new foods:** Be especially cautious if you have any medical conditions.

- **Share your knowledge:** Teach others how to forage safely and sustainably.

KITCHEN ESSENTIALS

You don't have to spend a fortune on specialist kitchenware; you can manage well with basic cooking utensils and a little ingenuity. A few large pans, a sieve and colander are all essential, and it's very useful to have some cotton muslin – although a clean cotton tea towel will work well, too. A pestle and mortar if you have one, or a food processor, will make life easier. Jam jars and bottles of differing sizes – new or recycled, as long as the lids are clean and undamaged – always look lovely with handwritten labels.

Carrier oils: You can use almond oil (avoid if you have a nut allergy), peach kernel oil or even olive oil. These are easily available online and in some health food shops.

How to sterilize jars and bottles:

1. Wash the jars and lids thoroughly in hot soapy water and rinse.

2. Lay the jars (without their lids) in an oven preheated to 140°C (285°F) for 10–15 minutes until dry.

3. Soak the lids in boiling water in a bowl, then dry thoroughly with kitchen paper before use.

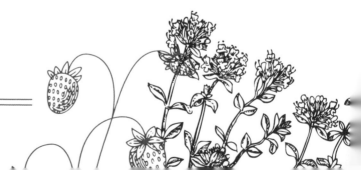

CONVERSIONS AND MEASUREMENTS

All the conversions in the tables below are close approximates which have been rounded up or down. When using a recipe, always stick to one unit of measurement and do not alternate between them.

LIQUID MEASUREMENTS

5 ml = 1 tsp
15 ml = 1 tbsp
30 ml = ⅛ cup
60 ml = ¼ cup
120 ml = ½ cup
240 ml = 1 cup
500 ml = 2¼ cups

DRIED INGREDIENT MEASUREMENTS

5 g = 1 tsp
15 g = 1 tbsp
30 g poppy seeds = ¼ cup
100 g caster sugar = ½ cup
300 g blackberries = 2 cups
400 g hazelnuts = 3 cups
450 g caster sugar = 2¼ cups

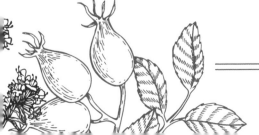

A BRIEF HISTORY OF "CUNNING FOLK"

Other names for cunning folk: wise woman/man, white witch, charmer, hedge witch, soothsayer

"Cunning folk" of some description could once be found in nearly every medieval settlement in Britain. These people were called upon to heal sickness in both humans and animals, to find and punish thieves, to help crops to grow, to look into the future, to cast horoscopes, to tell fortunes and to help people find love. Quite a job description! For their services, cunning folk often charged a small fee or accepted goods from the poor, and asked the gentry for a much higher price.

Though "black magic" was thought to come from the devil, the white magic practised by cunning folk was initially regarded by the Church as a "gift from the angels" and, as such, was considered beneficial. Cunning folk were the contemporary experts on preventative measures against black witchcraft and could offer a lot more help in this area than any physician or holy man. They not only offered protective charms and potions but could also identify and disarm a black witch by using counter-spells.

In 1644, Reverend William Brearley was lodging in a Suffolk village. His landlady had been ill for quite a while, and her husband was worried that she had been cursed. When a cunning man came knocking, her husband was advised by the cunning man to:

> *"Take a Bottle, and put his Wife's Urine into it, together with Pins and Needles and Nails, and Cork them up, and set the Bottle to the Fire, but be sure the Cork be fast in it, that it not fly out."*

Regrettably the cork did fly out and the counter magic was unsuccessful so, when the cunning man returned, he told the husband to "bury it in the Earth; and that will do the feat". After this, the wife soon recovered to full health.

An illustration of how popular cunning folk were viewed appears in a sermon in 1552 by Bishop Hugh Latimer:

"A great many of us when we be in trouble, or sickness, or lose anything, we run hither and thither to witches, or sorcerers, whom we call wise men... seeking aid and comfort at their hands."

Cunning folk rarely wrote their remedies down, although luckily some still survive, having been passed down orally. For example, a cure for thrush in children was recorded by John Aubrey in his book *Miscellanies*:

"Take a living frog, and hold it in a cloth, that it does not go down into the child's mouth; and put the head into the child's mouth 'till it is dead; and then take another frog and do the same."

And for toothache:

"Take a new nail, and make the gum bleed with it, and then drive it into an oak."

The educated classes did not always approve of the "gainful trade" of cunning folk and criticized and mocked them, even trying to enforce laws against them. In the sixteenth century across England, many people, mostly women, were accused of witchcraft by members of their local communities and put on trial; thankfully cunning folk rarely suffered this fate as their work was very much valued by the local community.

The Witchcraft Act of 1736 took the opinion that magic didn't exist, and that there had never been any "real" witches – an abrupt change from previous laws. This new act came down much more heavily on the cunning folk, who claimed that they performed genuine magical spells. It portrayed the cunning folk as practitioners of "explicitly fraudulent practices designed to fool the credulous" in order to profit from them. Anyone found guilty "faced a maximum sentence of one year's imprisonment without bail, and quarterly appearances in the pillory on market days".

Belief in supernatural powers slowly declined, especially among Puritan authors and more educated members of society. Cunning folk gradually began to be ridiculed and considered to be fraudsters by the villagers they had previously served, forcing many of them to stop practising. Sadly, the tradition of cunning folk eventually disappeared.

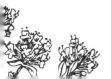

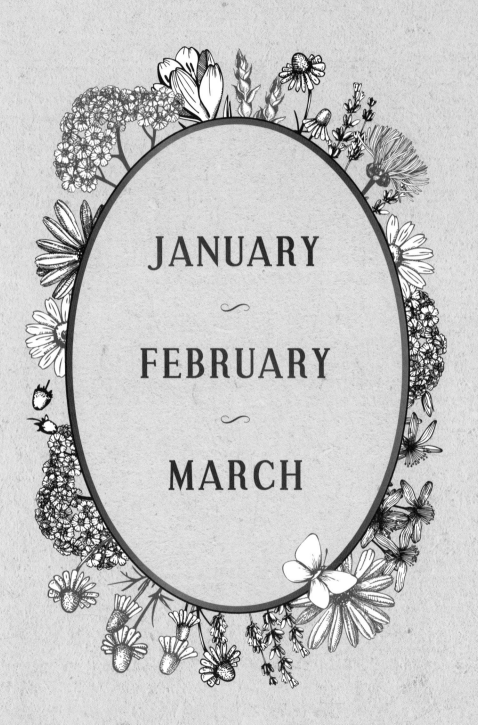

JANUARY

FEBRUARY

MARCH

Although you might not expect wild food to be in abundance at this time of year, you'll be surprised to learn that there are still some tasty greens and roots on offer. These are certainly quieter months in the foraging calendar, with the berries and nuts of autumn long gone, but even on the greyest of days in the depths of winter you'll still be able to discover some medicinal and foodie treasures.

In the northern hemisphere our ancestors would have foraged for nettles, chickweed, hairy bitter cress, common sorrel, wild chervil and dandelion roots to supplement their winter diet. These foraged greens were a vital supply of vitamins and minerals and would have been made into a "pottage" with whatever meat, vegetables and grains they had left from the autumn. Pottage was a thick soup or stew that was often kept going on the stove for several days and was a lifeline during the so-called "hungry gap" before the majority of crops were available later in the spring.

I like to spend the winter months clearing out my store cupboards and freezers and making lists of what needs using up before I even think of gathering more. Check any dried plant material to ensure that it is free from mould and still smells as it should. Prepare any infused oils and vinegars with last year's foraged goods so that you can start with a clean slate in the spring.

As the earth warms, garlic mustard, ground elder and the first tender shoots of delicious wild garlic will begin to appear, and you may find gorse flowers to add to your baking or for tea or syrup. It can still be chilly in March but this is officially the beginning of spring. Cleavers, also known as sticky weed, begin to appear. We all remember throwing this particular weed at our friends' jumpers with much hilarity during our schooldays, but it also has wonderful cleansing properties when added to a jug of cold water and drunk.

It is likely to be cold and damp when you head out, so wrap up warm, pull on your wellies and grab a basket. Don't forget your trowel if you're searching for roots or your gloves if you wish to pick nettle tops. Bring your *Hedgerow Apothecary Forager's Handbook* with you, and don't be too disappointed if you come home empty-handed – after all, you've benefitted from fresh air and exercise and rediscovered an important connection with nature.

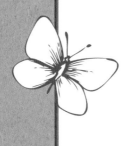

WHERE TO GO

The countryside, woodlands and vegetation or hedgerows along public footpaths are the obvious places to forage, but don't forget that parks, gardens and shorelines can reap rewards, too. If you live in the city, try to head for spaces away from busy roads and pollution. Explore the perimeter of your local park or canal towpath for treasures, avoiding popular dog-walking areas. Try to look for an area with lots of weeds, as this would indicate that your foraged finds are free from pesticides. Look out for common sorrel and garlic mustard in woodland, chickweed and dandelion root along field edges and verges and, of course, the ever-present nettles.

Examine your finds carefully once you get home and discard anything that isn't at its best. Give fruit a rinse before using and try to prepare it as soon as possible to avoid waste.

FOLKLORE AND TRADITIONS

JANUARY

Named after Janus – the Roman god of beginnings, transitions, duality, doors and gateways – January is the door to the New Year. It is traditional to kiss your love at the stroke of midnight to ensure continuing affection for the next twelve months. Failure to do so will have the opposite effect! Line up a dark-haired visitor to cross your threshold just after midnight: they should be carrying a piece of coal (to make sure that you are always warm), some bread (to keep you from going hungry), some money (for wealth) and some form of greenery (to ensure a long life).

DANDELION

The childhood joy of gently blowing the seeds off a dandelion globe can not only help you to tell the time, it can also tell you how much you are loved. Blow off all the seeds in one go and you are loved with a passion; however, if some seeds remain, your partner has some doubts, and if lots of seeds remain it might be best to look elsewhere for love. You can also blow the seeds in the direction of an absent love to send a message to them.

If all that wasn't enough, the dandelion globe can also predict the weather. In fine sunny weather the globe is round and fluffy. If rain is on its way, the globe shuts like an umbrella until the risk of rain has passed.

FEBRUARY

February is named after the ancient Roman festival of purification, *"februa"*, and reflects the rituals undertaken by our Roman ancestors in preparation for spring. The ancient festival of Candlemas on 2 February celebrates the return of the light and marks the midpoint between the shortest day and the spring equinox.

NETTLE

Nettles were used to thrash the devil out of poor souls believed to be possessed. It used to be believed that holding a nettle during a thunderstorm – if you could bear the stings – would prevent you from getting struck by lightning. Carrying yarrow with it was believed to help you become fearless, too – very useful during a thunderstorm, although I don't recommend that you try it!

MARCH

March was actually the start of the New Year for Romans, originally named *"Martius"* after Mars, the god of war. It was traditionally a time that military campaigns would resume after being interrupted by severe winter weather. It is also the month of the spring equinox, signifying the midpoint between winter and summer, when day and night are almost of equal length – also known as the start of spring.

WILD GARLIC

The plant's Latin name, *Allium ursinum*, literally means "bear garlic". This odd nickname comes from the belief that bears – as well as wild boar and badgers – ate wild garlic to regain their strength after a winter of hibernation.

Wild garlic was planted in the thatch of Irish cottages to ward off faeries and bring good luck. Roman soldiers heading to battle and athletes about to compete chewed a piece of wild garlic to give them strength for victory.

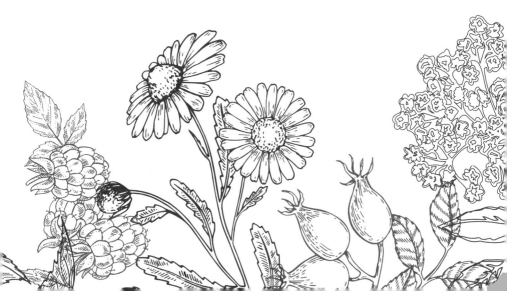

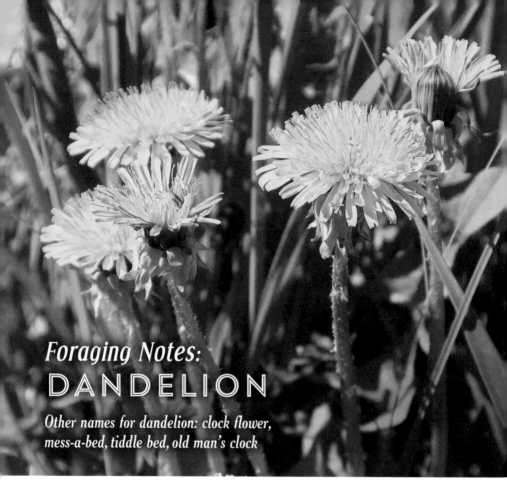

Foraging Notes:
DANDELION

Other names for dandelion: clock flower,
mess-a-bed, tiddle bed, old man's clock

HOW TO IDENTIFY: Probably the most familiar of UK wild flowers as it grows everywhere. The beautiful golden yellow flowers shine like little suns in the spring before turning to fluffy dandelion clocks later on in the summer.

The leaves are very distinctive, with "lion's tooth" (the French being *"dent-du-lion"*) edges. The stem is smooth and hollow and will ooze a milky sap once broken open.

COMMON USES: Dandelion is high in potassium and vitamins A, B, C and D, which can cleanse the blood and stimulate the liver. Young, tender leaves can be mixed into a green salad or made into pesto with pine nuts, olive oil and parmesan cheese. The flowers are traditionally made into wine, beer, cordials and vodka. The root, of course, is combined with burdock root to make a delicious tonic.

NOTES

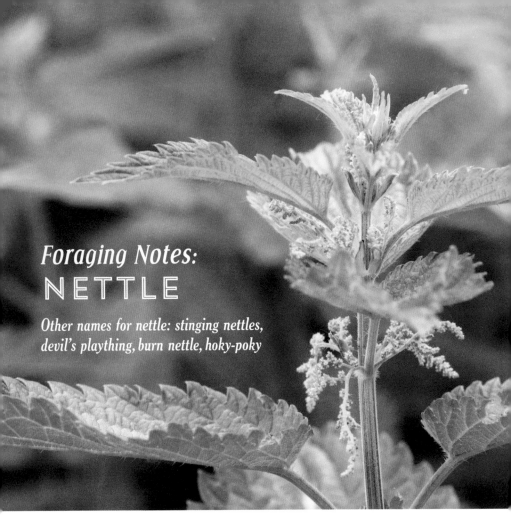

Foraging Notes:
NETTLE

*Other names for nettle: stinging nettles,
devil's plaything, burn nettle, hoky-poky*

HOW TO IDENTIFY: Nettles seemingly grow everywhere where there might be vulnerable bare arms and legs, and are often felt before they are seen! Dark green, hairy, heart-shaped stinging leaves are arranged in pairs along a tall, straight stem. The flowers form at the base of the leaves and are greenish-white with yellow anthers.

COMMON USES: Full of vitamins, protein and iron, nettles make a useful substitute for spinach in cooking, a cleansing tea and a tasty nutrient-packed soup – don't worry, the stings completely disappear after cooking.

Today, the chlorophyll of nettle is used as a green dye and is known as the food colourant E140.

NOTES

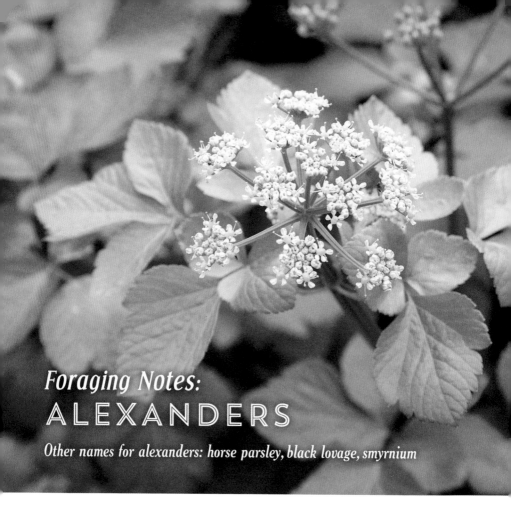

Foraging Notes:
ALEXANDERS

Other names for alexanders: horse parsley, black lovage, smyrnium

HOW TO IDENTIFY: Grows up to 1.5 m tall with bright green-toothed leaves arranged in threes. It has a thick juicy stem that resembles celery, with greenish-yellow umbrella-shaped flowers that smell spicy and sweet. Alexanders can be found at the edges of woodlands, in coastal areas and along river banks.

COMMON USES: Originally brought to Europe by the Romans to use as a pot-herb, alexanders are commonly found in towns and cities that were once under Roman rule. The leaves, stems and flowers are all edible and have a flavour similar to celery or parsley. You can add them to soups and stews. Wash and trim young stems, steam for 5–10 minutes until tender, then serve with a knob of butter and a squeeze of lime juice.

NOTES

Foraging Notes:
VIOLET

Other names for violet: sweet violet,
blue violet, English violet

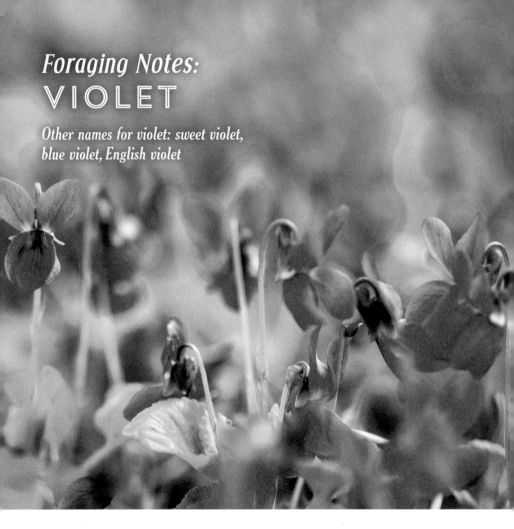

HOW TO IDENTIFY: Violets grow on shaded banks, under hedges and in woodland. The pansy-like flowers appear from late March to early April and are not always violet in colour – they can be white, pink or dark indigo blue. If you've ever eaten Parma Violet sweets, then you'll have a good idea of what the flowers taste like. The heart-shaped leaves are slightly downy and start off bright green, turning darker as they age.

COMMON USES: Violets have been a popular flavour and scent for many centuries. Today they are used to flavour sweets and chocolates, as well as to fragrance perfumes, soaps and cosmetics. They can also be sewn into small sachets to aid a good night's sleep when placed under your pillow.

NOTES

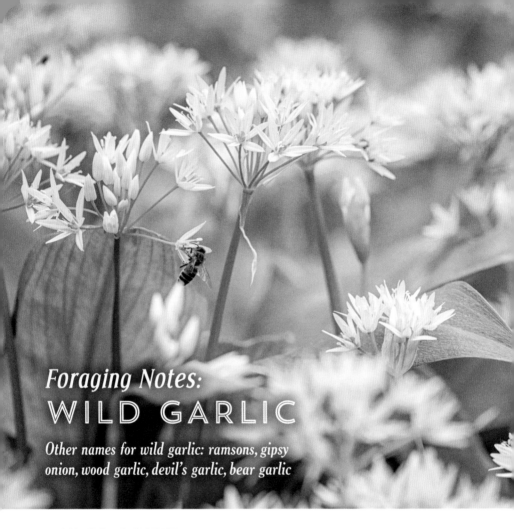

Foraging Notes:
WILD GARLIC

Other names for wild garlic: ramsons, gipsy onion, wood garlic, devil's garlic, bear garlic

HOW TO IDENTIFY: Wild garlic grows in damp, ancient woodlands and has a very distinctive, garlicky smell. Be careful when foraging for wild garlic as the leaves look very similar to lily of the valley and lords-and-ladies, both of which are poisonous. Crush the leaves and sniff them for that pungent garlic smell. Its broad, spear-like leaves appear in early March, followed by a profusion of starry white flowers carpeting the woodland floor.

COMMON USES: Leaves, bulbs and flowers are all edible, adding a subtle garlic flavour to food. Similar in taste to chives, the young, tender leaves can be used in salads and sauces, added to scrambled eggs or omelettes, stirred into risottos, or, my favourite way to use them – pesto (see page 39).

NOTES

OTHER FORAGING FINDS

CHICKWEED

Growing just a few inches off the ground, this plant thrives in cool, damp conditions. It has five star-like petals and small teardrop-shaped leaves along its stem. Bursting in iron, manganese, zinc and vitamins A, D and B, chickweed is a great substitute for spinach – perfect in a salad or homemade pesto. The leaves also have soothing properties and can be used in a poultice to ease chilblains, eczema and insect stings.

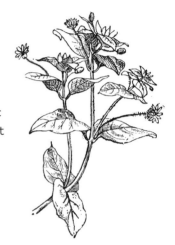

WOOD SORREL

Known for its delicate five-petalled white flowers tinged with pink or purple veining, wood sorrel has three heart-shaped leaves similar in shape to clover. It likes to grow in damp shady places such as hedgerows and woodlands and can be seen in flower between Easter and Whitsun (traditionally celebrated seven Sundays after Easter Sunday).

In the Middle Ages the delicate plant was so popular as an ingredient in soups, salads and spinach that it was widely cultivated in England. For a long time wood sorrel was a source of oxalic acid, used in textile dyeing as a cleaning agent to remove ink and rust stains. It was also used to bleach straw and stearin for soap- and candle-making and to clean copper and brass.

The leaves, stems and flowers are all edible, but eat it in moderation as, like many leafy greens, the oxalic acid could give you an upset stomach. (Not recommended for anyone with kidney stones or gout.)

CROW GARLIC

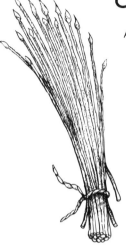

A bulb-forming variety of wild onion with slender, hollow leaves similar to chives, which sometimes grows in a delightfully twisted fashion. You may be lucky enough to find crow garlic growing in grassland, hedgerows, meadows and along coastal paths. It is hated by farmers as large amounts growing in pasture can alter the taste of the milk yield. The leaves can be used in similar ways to chives and the bulbs, although small and tricky to peel, can be added to cooking as a garlic substitute.

As with other members of the onion family, crow garlic is toxic to dogs and can cause anaemia, so keep it away from your canine companions.

GROUND ELDER

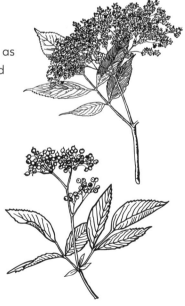

Originally brought to Europe by the Romans as a food staple, ground elder is now considered to be a nuisance to gardeners as it can form a suffocating green carpet very quickly. The toothed leaves are arranged in groups of three, at the end of leaf stems with small clusters of white flowers. You'll find it growing in abundance in woodlands, alongside waterways and on waste ground. It was another popular addition to medieval pottage and can be eaten cooked or raw as a spinach substitute – it is similarly high in vitamin C.

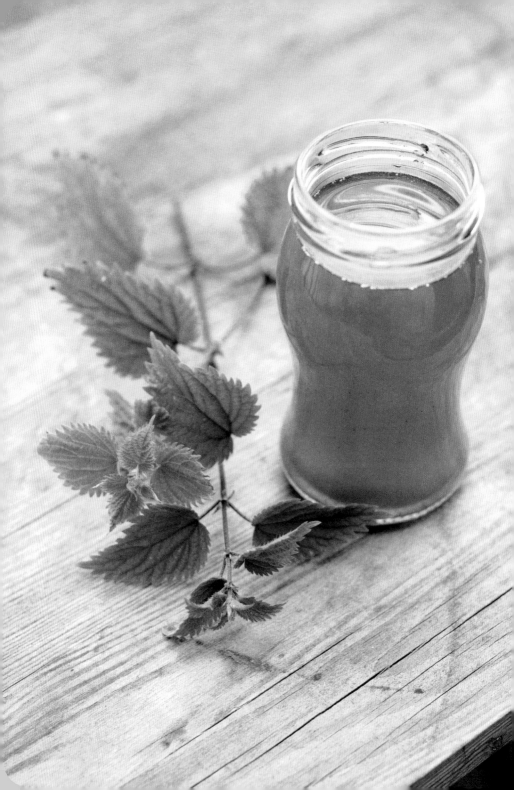

NETTLE HAIR TONIC

Use as a final rinse to stimulate hair growth and strengthen the hair. Remember to wear long sleeves and gloves to gather your nettles, and forage away from popular dog-walking areas.

Makes enough for two applications on short hair or one application for longer hair

INGREDIENTS

1 large bunch of fresh nettle tops

500 ml water

500 ml white wine (or apple cider) vinegar

1 tbsp of chopped fresh herbs or 1 tsp dried herbs of your choice (sage or rosemary for dark hair, camomile or sunflower petals for fair hair, calendula or marigold for red hair)

Essential oils (optional)

METHOD

Put the nettles in a large pan with the water and vinegar and bring to a simmer for 2 hours.

Stir in the herbs; essential oils could be added, too.

Allow the liquid to cool.

Strain through muslin and bottle.

Use within one week.

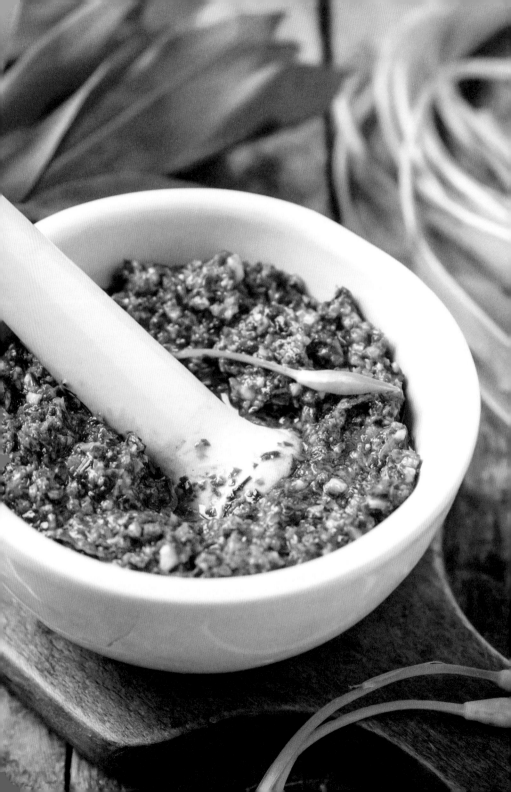

WILD GARLIC PESTO

Pesto is pretty much raw when eaten, keeping all the valuable antiviral, antibiotic and antibacterial properties and vitamins of the ingredients intact. Pick young, tender garlic leaves away from busy roads and dog-walkers.

Makes one jar

INGREDIENTS

Handful of well-washed young wild garlic leaves

Handful of basil leaves

Olive oil

200 g finely grated parmesan cheese (or dairy-free alternative)

150 g pine nuts (or walnuts), roughly chopped

Salt to taste

METHOD

Blend the wild garlic and basil in a pestle and mortar or food processor with enough olive oil to make a smooth paste.

Stir in the cheese and nuts. Season to taste.

Stir through freshly cooked pasta, knead into bread dough or slip under the skin of a chicken before roasting.

Store any leftover pesto in the fridge in an airtight container and use within three days.

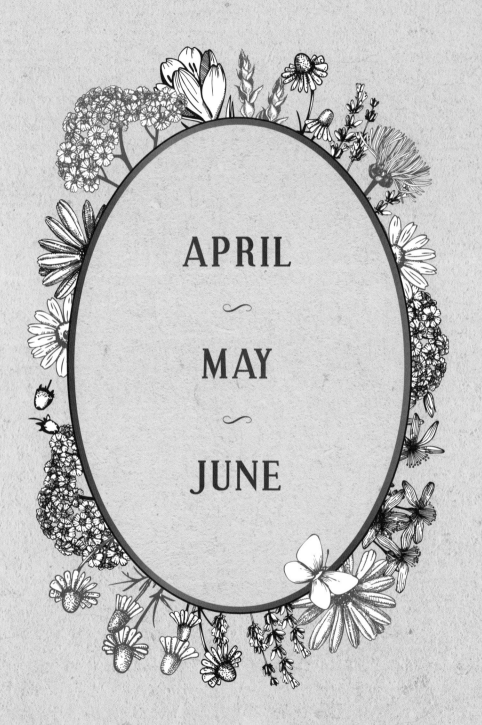

APRIL

MAY

JUNE

After the long dark days of winter, spring is now well underway; the sun is slowly warming the soil, the days are getting longer and everything is bursting back to life. You only have to look to your own back garden or local park to gauge the soil temperature; if the weeds are growing, the free edibles and medicines will be emerging, too. Native wildlife is busy with nest building, birdsong fills the air and the urge for us to venture outside grows ever stronger.

Spring has long been seen as a season of new beginnings, offering up the hope of fresh food in abundance after the fallow winter months. In the Middle Ages, spring was the time for our ancestors to fling open the doors and window shutters after a long winter confined in a smoky environment among people and smelly animals. They had survived all winter on salted and smoked meat with very few fresh vegetables, so spring was a very busy time not just for foraging and planting, but also for lambing and calving. Herbs, nuts, flowers and roots were all foraged by poorer members of society to supplement a meagre diet of oats, cabbage, beans and bread made from rye, millet and barley grains.

You should start to see the appearance of flowers on blackthorn as well as hawthorn and wild cherry blossom. Cow parsley begins to line the edges of country lanes and nettles, cowslips, primroses, wild violets, yellow gorse flowers and forget-me-nots all appear in the grass verges and fields.

If wild garlic is now in bloom the leaves may be too tough to use, but the starry white flowers can still give a gentle garlic flavour to salads. Dandelion leaves, roots and flowers are edible and the blooms can be infused into carrier oil

41

to make a soothing muscle rub or turned into natural sunscreen along with the addition of zinc oxide and coconut oil (see page 73) – good preparation for the summer months, and it will keep in the fridge for a year.

It's worth looking back at your notes on where you found good foraging land and the useful species that were growing there. Revisit them and see what else you can discover and how the landscape has changed. Keep a lookout for the creamy blossoms of elderflower along the hedgerow, which is useful for skincare and cordial. Remember that if you pick the blossoms, you'll be sacrificing some berries in the autumn.

Spring is a busy time for farmers and it's really important that you don't trespass into fields of pregnant cattle or sheep, especially if you have a canine companion with you. Crops are also very small and vulnerable at this time of year so avoid straying from the footpaths and ALWAYS follow the country code.

As Thomas Tusser, a sixteenth-century farmer and poet, reminds us, "Sweet April showers, do spring May flowers," so don't discard the waterproofs and wellies just yet.

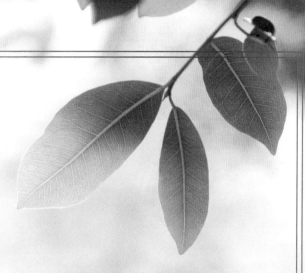

WHERE TO GO

Most people think of the foraging season being from August to October, but spring really is the start of the wild food harvest and you'll start to see young buds appearing all around now. If you're new to foraging, why not take a spring walk around your local park or open space and see what you can identify? Make notes about what you see. Foraging finds can pop up in the most unexpected places, so keep those eyes open. Hedgerows will slowly come to life with hawthorn blossom followed by elderflower, and the woodland floor will soon be covered in wild garlic as the tree canopy bursts into a hundred different shades of green.

FOLKLORE AND TRADITIONS

APRIL

The word "April" comes from the Latin *"aperire"* meaning "to open". This month is the start of the growing season and everything is beginning to open.

The tradition of April Fool's Day is believed to have come to the UK from France or Germany in the mid-seventeenth century. Originally it was purely for the amusement of adults who would try to trick others into going on "fool's errands" for non-existent objects such as "pigeon milk", and has carried on well into the twenty-first century with errands for items like "tartan paint". Make sure that you play your trick before midday, otherwise "April fool is gone and past, You're the biggest fool at last!"

COW PARSLEY

Frothy cow parsley lines the edges of country lanes. It was historically called "mother dies" or "kill your mother quick" to discourage children from picking it and bringing it home as they may accidentally pick the very similar – yet highly poisonous – hemlock.

MAY

May takes its name from the Roman goddess Maia, who is associated with fertility and growth. May Day or Beltane was celebrated by our pagan ancestors as the first day of summer with the return of the sun and fertility to the soil.

It's especially important for young ladies to rise early on May Day if they wish to take advantage of the magic of this old rhyme:

"The fair maid who,
the first of May, goes to the fields at the break of day,
and washes in dew from the hawthorn tree,
will ever after handsome be."

HAWTHORN

An infusion of hawthorn flowers and leaves was used to treat sore throats, while chewing the bark gave relief from toothache. One folkloric cure for warts tells the sufferer to rub a live slug over their warts then impale the poor creature on the spikes of a hawthorn tree. As the slug shrivels and dies, the warts will, too.

JUNE

The month of June is believed to be named after the Roman goddess Juno, who was the wife of Jupiter and the goddess of women and marriage.

The summer solstice occurs between 20 and 22 June and marks midsummer, the longest day and the shortest night. Our Celtic ancestors celebrated by lighting bonfires to add to the sun's energy and wore garlands of protective herbs to ward off evil spirits that appeared on this day.

ELDER

You'll see the creamy-white sprays of elderflowers dominating the hedgerows at the moment. Pick a few to turn into cordial but also make a note of where they are in your handbook so that you can return at the end of summer to gather elderberries for rob (see page 121).

An elder tree that has self-seeded in your garden was said to prevent evil spirits, negative influences and lightning from entering the home, and one planted by a cowshed was believed to protect your cattle.

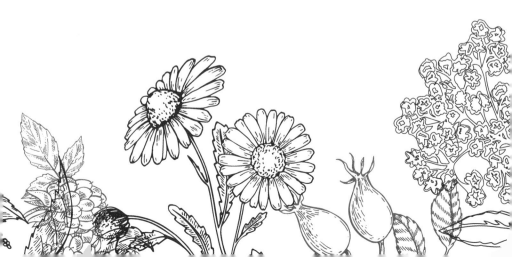

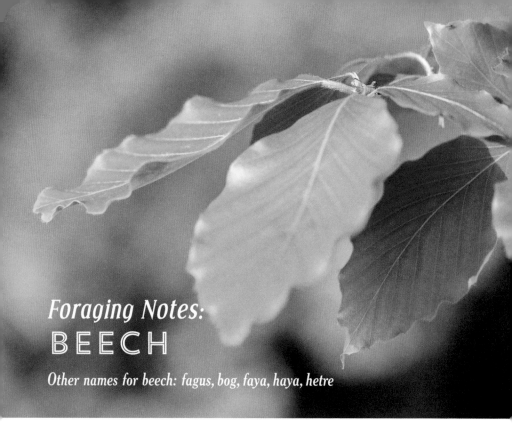

Foraging Notes:
BEECH

Other names for beech: fagus, bog, faya, haya, hetre

HOW TO IDENTIFY: Commonly found growing on chalky soil and beside hedgerows, the elegant beech is surely one of the UK's most graceful native trees. It grows to approximately 40 m (130 ft) tall and is memorable for its large dome-shaped crown and smooth grey bark.

Beech leaves in the spring are soft, smooth and diaphanous, with a delicious lime-green hue. By summer, the oval leaves have changed to dark green and the silky hairs seen on the young leaves have disappeared. Autumn's chill turns the leaves a striking copper colour, catching the fading light in the hedgerows and woodlands. Male and female flowers grow on the same tree in spring, the male producing catkins while the female flowers make way for beech nuts in autumn.

COMMON USES: Beech wood burns well and is traditionally used to smoke herring. Beech nuts are normally fed to pigs but can be roasted for a healthy human snack or ground to use as a coffee substitute. Beech trees make a beautiful hedging plant that changes colour with the seasons.

NOTES

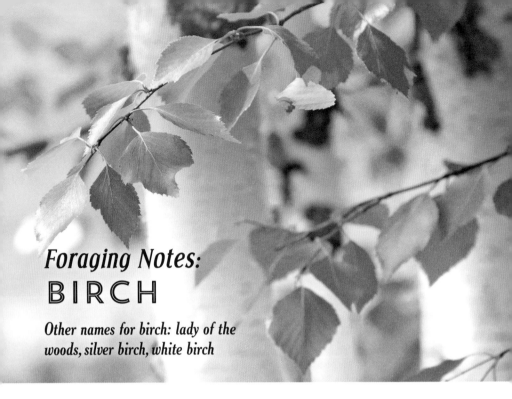

Foraging Notes:
BIRCH

Other names for birch: lady of the woods, silver birch, white birch

HOW TO IDENTIFY: With its beautiful silvery-white tissue-paper bark and elegant drooping branches, the birch has a light canopy that allows dappled shade to reach the woodland floor. The leaves are small, pale green and triangular, with jagged edges that fade to yellow in the autumn. Attractive yellow catkins appear in spring, changing to dark red with masses of seeds to be distributed on the breeze in autumn.

COMMON USES: Birch sap was prized for its sticky, sweet, delicate flavour, which must have been very welcome to our ancestors after a long winter of very bland food. Tapping is done in early spring using a mature birch tree. With a sterile drill bit, drill a hole about 1 m (3 ft) from the ground, angling the drill slightly upward – the hole should be about 5 mm (¼ in.) in diameter. Insert some sterile tubing into the hole and catch the sap in a clean container as it flows out. Don't be greedy – only take what you need, then gently remove the tubing and press on the wound until it stops flowing. The sap doesn't stay fresh for long, so use it quickly to make wine, syrup or a soothing skin wash.

Only drill into birch trees if they are on your land or with the permission of the landowner.

NOTES

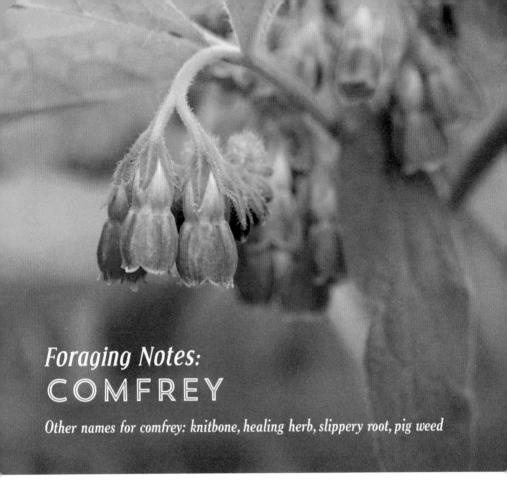

Foraging Notes:
COMFREY

Other names for comfrey: knitbone, healing herb, slippery root, pig weed

HOW TO IDENTIFY: Comfrey grows in damp, shady woodlands and hedgerows. It is quite easy to spot with its broad, lance-shaped hairy leaves, which look similar to foxglove leaves (comfrey leaves have smooth edges while the leaves of the foxglove are finely toothed). Be careful as this can fool novice foragers, with deadly consequences, as foxglove leaves are toxic! Clusters of pink, purple or white trumpet-shaped flowers begin to appear in May, dangling on the end of thick, hairy stems.

COMMON USES: Comfrey leaves can easily be made into a potassium-rich fertilizer to benefit your home-grown fruit and flowers. Smallholders value comfrey leaves as a natural supply of protein for their cattle and chickens.

Using comfrey internally is NOT recommended unless prescribed by a qualified herbalist.

NOTES

Foraging Notes:
DAISY

Other names for daisy: day's eyes, lawn daisy, bruisewort, child's flower

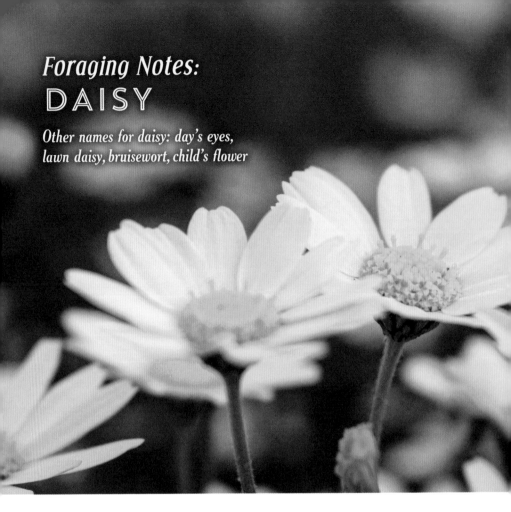

HOW TO IDENTIFY: Commonly found in lawns and grassy areas. These tiny yellow-centred flowers have pretty white petals which are often tipped with pink.

COMMON USES: Daisy flowers and leaves are edible and can be added to salads, although they have a somewhat bitter taste. With anti-inflammatory, wound-healing and pain-relieving properties similar to arnica, daisies can be infused into carrier oil to make a soothing balm.

Allow daisies to wilt overnight, then place in a jam jar and cover with 100 ml of carrier oil (almond, peach kernel or sunflower). Cover the jar and leave on a sunny windowsill for two weeks, then strain. Heat the oil in a bain-marie with 10 g of beeswax, then pour into clean tins or jars.

NOTES

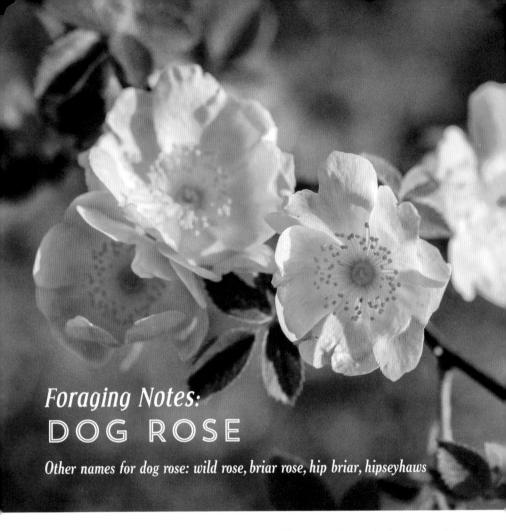

Foraging Notes:
DOG ROSE

Other names for dog rose: wild rose, briar rose, hip briar, hipseyhaws

HOW TO IDENTIFY: A distinctive rambling, sturdy shrub that scrambles through country hedgerows. The tall, arching stems are covered in curved thorns with dark-green, oval-toothed leaves. It produces delicate five-petalled flowers in pink or white from June to July, followed by bright red hips, which light up the autumn hedgerows.

COMMON USES: The delicate petals of the dog rose can be crystallized by painting them with beaten egg white and then dipping them in sugar to make beautiful edible cake decorations. Rosehips appear later in the autumn, so keep note of where you have found dog rose plants to enable you to return and pick some for rosehip syrup.

NOTES

Foraging Notes:
ELDER

*Other names for elder: devil's wood,
old gal, dog tree, Judas tree*

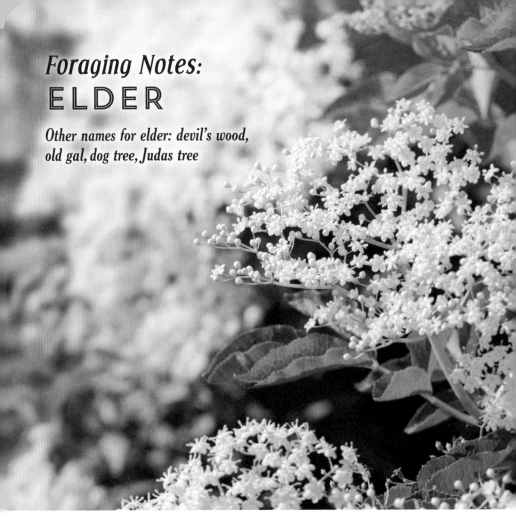

HOW TO IDENTIFY: Common in hedgerows and woods, this small tree has a corky bark that splits as it matures. The leaves comprise five to seven oval leaflets with feathery edges. Clusters of fragrant creamy white flowers appear in summer followed by small dark purple berries in the autumn.

COMMON USES: Elderberries are full of antioxidants and vitamin C and can be turned into an effective home remedy for coughs, colds and sore throats (see page 121).

An English summer wouldn't be the same without a fragrant glass of elderflower cordial in the sunshine. The cordial can also be drizzled over cakes and pancakes and makes a gin and tonic very special indeed!

NOTES

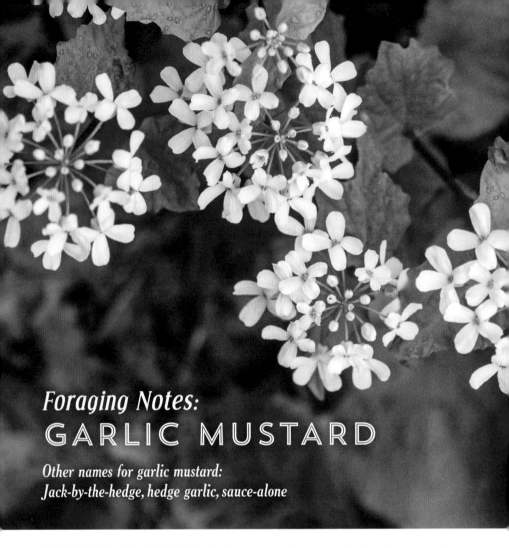

Foraging Notes:
GARLIC MUSTARD

Other names for garlic mustard:
Jack-by-the-hedge, hedge garlic, sauce-alone

HOW TO IDENTIFY: Garlic mustard enjoys shady places such as hedgerows and the edges of woodland. It grows to about 1 m (3 ft) tall, with hairless heart-shaped leaves and small white flowers. Crush the leaves and you will release a distinctly garlicky scent.

COMMON USES: The leaves of garlic mustard can be used to flavour fish or meat, and fresh young leaves are a delicious addition to salads. Pull up the roots, give them a scrub, chop them up in a food processor and you'll have a super-spicy sauce similar to horseradish.

Roots should only be dug up with the permission of the landowner.

NOTES

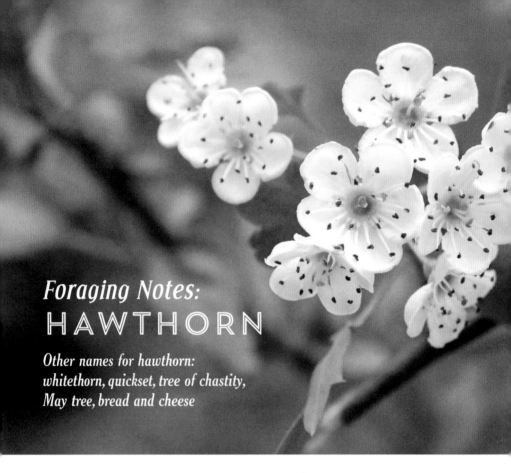

Foraging Notes:
HAWTHORN

Other names for hawthorn:
whitethorn, quickset, tree of chastity,
May tree, bread and cheese

HOW TO IDENTIFY: Found growing in most hedgerows, the hawthorn has small, deep-lobed leaves that look almost divided. Young stems are reddish in colour with sharp thorns, hence the name. In spring it is covered in an abundance of delicate white flowers known as "May blossom" and these turn into dark, berry-like fruits known as "haws" in the autumn.

COMMON USES: Adding haws to other hedgerow fruit makes a delicious fruity jelly (similar to jam, but with the pips and skin removed).

   Modern medicine has recognized that haws have considerable benefits to heart health. They have been found to lower blood pressure, open the arteries and strengthen the heart.

*It is important not to take hawthorn without the advice of a qualified medical practitioner if you use beta blockers and other heart drugs.

NOTES

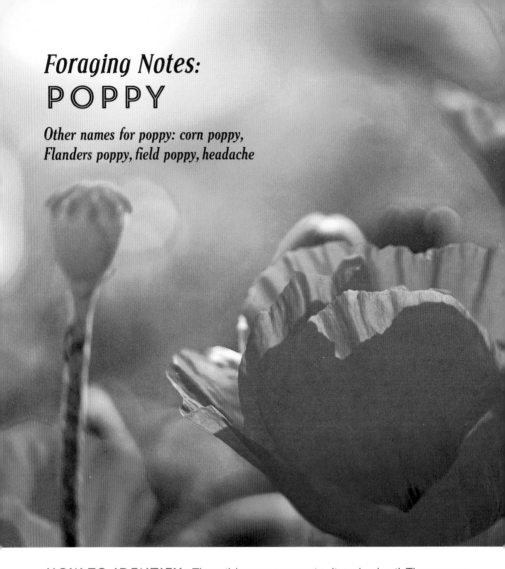

Foraging Notes:
POPPY

*Other names for poppy: corn poppy,
Flanders poppy, field poppy, headache*

HOW TO IDENTIFY: The wild poppy grows in disturbed soil. The papery thin scarlet flower barely lasts a day on its tall hairy stem.

COMMON USES: Red poppy petals can be used to brighten up your salad, and the seeds are delicious baked into cakes and bread. The tiny poppy seeds can be used as a gentle exfoliator to help give your skin a natural glow (see page 75). The petals and seeds are known to have mild sedative properties that were used to good effect by tired land girls and exhausted mothers during World War Two.

NOTES

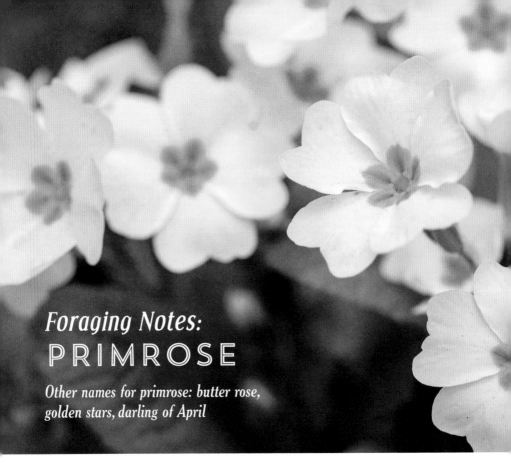

Foraging Notes:
PRIMROSE

*Other names for primrose: butter rose,
golden stars, darling of April*

HOW TO IDENTIFY: This pretty woodland perennial heralds the start of spring. It grows in neat clumps with pale lemon flowers dotted with a deeper yellow or orange centre. The single flowers have five notched petals on upright furry stalks. The crinkly, wrinkly, short-stemmed leaves have hairy undersides that form a rosette at the base of the plant.

COMMON USES: The flowers have been used to make a country wine, but as this uses very many flowers I feel this recipe is best left to the history books.

Primrose and other edible flowers such as viola can be crystallized to make delightful cake decorations. Simply paint the flowers very gently with beaten egg white (or aquafaba for a vegan option) then carefully cover in granulated sugar. Place the flower face down onto greaseproof paper and allow to dry for a day or two. Use immediately or store in an airtight container in a dry, dark place for up to six months.

NOTES

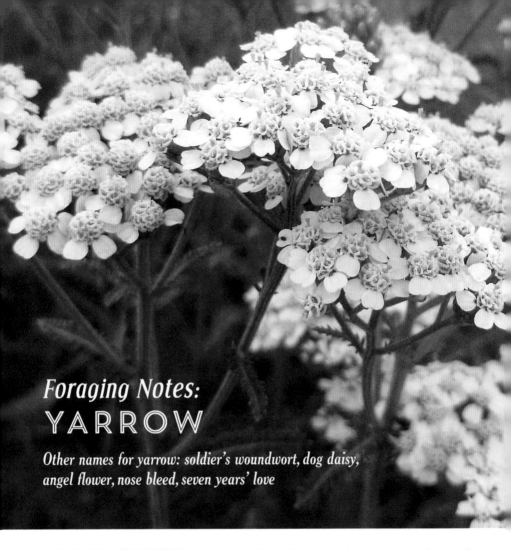

Foraging Notes:
YARROW

Other names for yarrow: soldier's woundwort, dog daisy,
angel flower, nose bleed, seven years' love

HOW TO IDENTIFY: Yarrow is found in abundance in grassland all over Britain. This ferny-leaved perennial can grow up to 1 m (3 ft) tall. The plant forms clumps that can be quite invasive, with long, straight stalks and feathery leaves, and white or pink flowers at the top. Crush the leaves and you will release its strong aroma.

COMMON USES: Yarrow is a useful herb to hang in your wardrobe as it deters insects. It was a popular vegetable in the seventeenth century; the young leaves were cooked like spinach or put into soup. The leaves can also be dried and used as a cooking herb.

NOTES

OTHER FORAGING FINDS

BORAGE

Borage is easily identified by its beautiful blue star-shaped flowers, which are thought to have been the inspiration for the colour of the Virgin Mary's robes in Renaissance paintings.

Its name comes from the Gaelic word *"borrach"* meaning "courage". Interestingly, modern research has discovered that borage increases the body's production of adrenalin when ingested.

Young borage leaves are cooling and soothing. Simply steep the leaves in boiled water, allow to cool and soak cotton pads in the solution and apply to the eyelids to help reduce the puffiness of tired eyes. Borage flowers look beautiful frozen into ice cubes to drop into a jug of Pimm's in the summer, and they can also be added to salads or crystallized to decorate cakes.

WILD THYME

A low-growing woody herb with a distinctive square stem marking it out as a member of the mint family. Small fragrant oval leaves and tiny purplish-pink flowers form dense mats that creep over chalk grasslands, cliffs and rocky places.

Faeries are said to love to inhabit the twisted and knotted branches of wild thyme, making it unlucky to bring into the house for fear of upsetting the fae. Thymol is a powerful antiseptic derived from thyme, and this can be found in mouthwash, hand sanitizer and acne medication.

GORSE

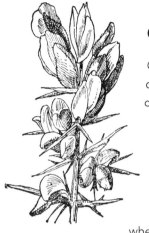

Gorse flourishes in poor soils like wasteland, shingle and the edges of grasslands and forests, and is one of the very rare plants that can carry blooms all year round.

Beware: gorse has edible yellow flowers, but it also has needle-sharp leaves! This made it a useful barrier for our ancestors, who used it to keep their livestock in and predators out.

The pea-like yellow flowers smell distinctly of coconut when warmed by the sun – some people say that they taste of coconut or almonds. Pop the flowers into salads for a burst of colour or infuse them into warm sugar syrup to pour over desserts and ice cream.

PIGNUTS

By the shape of its small delicate leaves, you may recognise pignuts as a member of the carrot family. It grows to around 40 cm (16 in.) in woodlands and hedgerows and is topped with clusters of umbrella-shaped flowers that appear between May and June. These will lead you to a small edible tuber, called a pignut, buried underground – a favourite treat for wild boar and badgers.

The tubers can be cleaned and eaten raw or roasted in the oven with a little oil. The taste has been compared to hazelnuts or sweet chestnuts, with a radish-like aftertaste.

As these need to be dug up it's important to get permission from the landowner before you forage for pignuts.

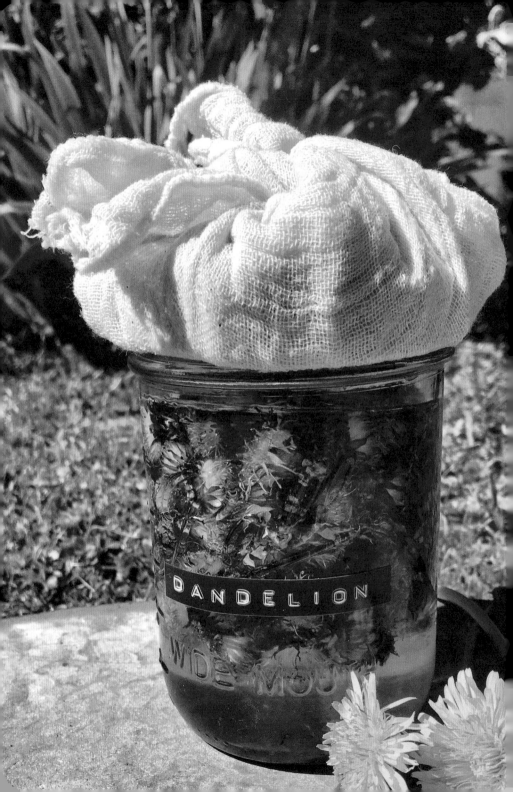

DANDELION-INFUSED OIL

This oil harnesses the wonderful anti-inflammatory properties of the humble dandelion flower to relax overused muscles and stiff necks. Dandelion offers natural sun protection, making this oil perfect to use as the base for dandelion sunscreen (see page 73). As always, gather your blossoms from an area that is free from dog-walkers and pesticides. Keeps for about a year.

YOU WILL NEED

Glass jar

Enough dandelion flowers to fill your glass jar

Carrier oil such as olive oil or almond oil

Muslin square

Storage jar(s)

METHOD

Pick your dandelions on a dry day and allow to wilt on kitchen towel out of direct sunlight for 24 hours to release excess moisture.

Once they are dry, fill a glass jar with the blossoms.

Top up the jar with olive oil, making sure that there are no air bubbles.

Secure the muslin square on top of the jar with twine or a rubber band and leave on a sunny windowsill for two weeks.

Pour your dandelion-infused oil through a fine sieve, catching the oil in a measuring jug.

Squeeze out as much oil as you can, then compost the blossoms.

Pour your oil into storage jar (or jars).

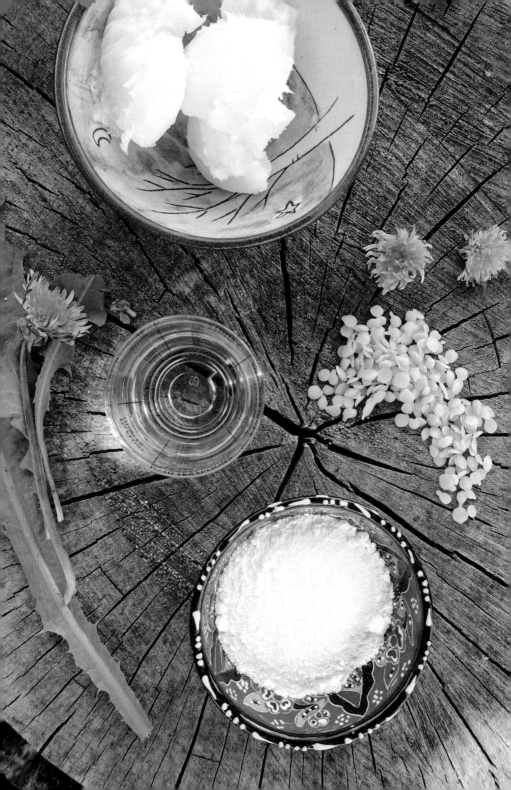

DANDELION SUNSCREEN

This sunscreen can provide protection from both UVA and UVB radiation. Unlike commercial brands, the SPF cannot be accurately calculated so please use cautiously.

Dandelion oil has a natural SPF of approximately 8 and coconut oil an SPF of around 7.

The more zinc oxide that you add, the higher the SPF, but the texture of your sunscreen will become more paste-like. Always buy "non-nano" zinc oxide powder as this will sit on top of your skin, helping to scatter the sun's rays.

Makes about 120 ml

INGREDIENTS

4 tbsp dandelion-infused oil (see page 71)

4 tbsp organic coconut oil

2 tbsp natural beeswax pellets

Zinc oxide powder – available from online retailers – for approximate SPF protection:

 SPF 6–11 = add 1 tbsp

 SPF 12–19 = add 1.5 tbsp

 SPF 20+ = add 2 tbsp

METHOD

Add the dandelion oil, coconut oil and beeswax to a heatproof bowl, place over a pan of boiling water and stir until melted.

Take the mixture off the heat and allow to cool slightly.

Sieve in your desired amount of zinc oxide and whisk thoroughly until cooled.

Pour into tins or jars and label.

Will keep for about a year. Keeping your sunscreen in the fridge will increase its shelf life.

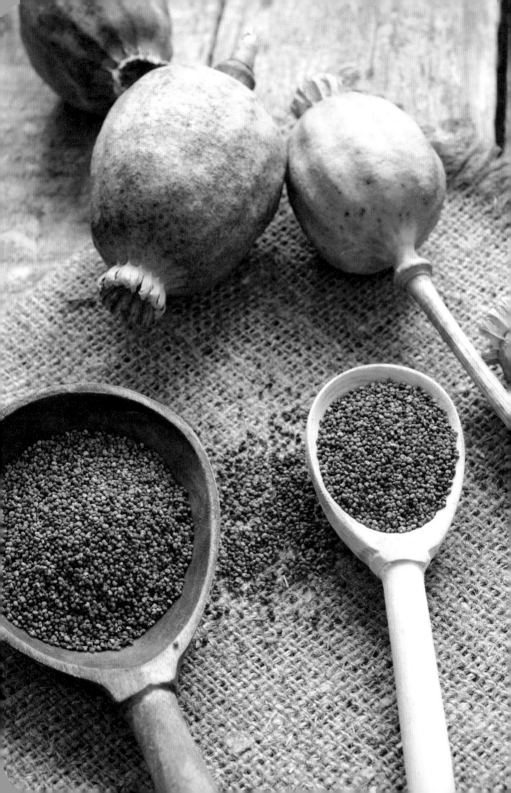

POPPY SEED FACIAL SCRUB

The essential fatty acids and antioxidants in poppy seeds help to give skin a natural glow. Lemon juice is antibacterial and can reduce redness and brighten the complexion.

Makes approximately 180 g

INGREDIENTS

100 g caster sugar

30 g poppy seeds

Finely grated zest from one unwaxed lemon

50 g coconut oil

2 tsp lemon juice

METHOD

Mix the sugar, poppy seeds and lemon zest together.

Gently melt the coconut oil and pour into the sugar mixture, add the lemon juice and combine.

The mixture should resemble wet sand.

Rub a small amount between the palms and gently apply to wet skin using a circular motion.

Rinse and pat dry.

Use within one month.

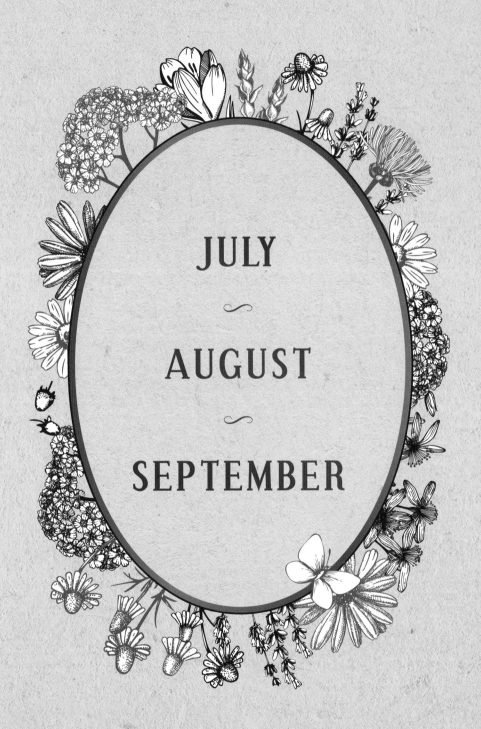

JULY

AUGUST

SEPTEMBER

During the summertime it was crucial that our ancestors made preparations for the lean winter months ahead. Meat or fish was covered in salt to draw out any moisture and kill bacteria, and was then hung in the rafters above a smoky fire. Vegetables could also be salted, dried or smoked, or pickled in the same way as many people still do today.

The hedgerows are now bursting with blossom from hawthorn, crab apple, blackthorn, bramble and wild rose, with a complementary understory of corn cockle, daisies, dandelion, ragged robin and lots, lots more. A small wildflower guide, along with your hedgerow guide, will give you hours of fun identifying the floral finds at this time of year. Make some notes, perhaps sketch a few specimens and take photos rather than picking the flowers – let's leave those for the pollinators.

This is the season of wildflower meadows, which look spectacular and are well worth seeking out. Many farmers now grow wildflower meadows around the edges of their land to provide a vital habitat for insects and those that feed on them. The farmer benefits from integrated pollination and pest control, the wildlife benefits from valuable nesting and foraging areas, and we benefit from the visual spectacle of a wildflower meadow.

Always check that you have right of way before wandering onto farmland and be respectful of any crops. Ordnance Survey provide up-to-date maps of public footpaths and bridleways both online and in print, with public footpaths clearly marked to guide you on your journey.

Your safety is vital, so never disturb livestock, especially if they are in calf or with young. Keep dogs on leads and always close gates behind you. Remember to "Respect, protect, enjoy" our wonderful countryside.

Towards the end of summer the hawthorn flowers will begin to produce red berries called haws; keep an eye out for these as they are a useful addition to hedgerow preserves and remedies in the autumn. Make a note in your hedgerow guide of the location of blackthorn, elder and wild rose, too – you'll need these for sloe gin (page 132), sloe port (page 147), elderberry rob (page 121) and rosehip syrup. It's important to use your guide to make notes on the progress of the hedgerow – some years I've been foraging for elder well into September, and other years they've gone over (or been eaten by the birds) before the end of August. Nature doesn't run to a strict timetable; keep an eye on how berries are progressing to avoid disappointment.

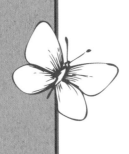

WHERE TO GO

Summer gives us the opportunity to forage a little further afield as the warm dry days and the promise of a picnic lunch with fresh leaves and berries might encourage you to walk for a little longer. Blackberries are now beginning to ripen, ready to be made into vinegar, crumble and jam. Dandelion leaves, garlic mustard and sheep's sorrel can all be gathered from woodland or fields to add to a tasty salad back at home. Public footpaths often take you through ancient woodlands and hedgerows – make notes in your handbook for future reference. Towpaths, embankments and cycle paths can all provide rich pickings but, as always, avoid busy roads, dog-walking areas and agricultural fields where pesticides have been used.

FOLKLORE AND TRADITIONS

JULY

July was originally known as *"Quintilis"* (meaning "fifth", as it was originally the fifth month, until the adoption of the Gregorian calendar in the sixteenth century turned it into the seventh) in ancient Rome, but was renamed in 44 BCE by the senate in honour of Julius Caesar who was born in this month.

Saint Swithin's Day falls on 15 July every year and folklore tells us that if it rains on this day, it will be wet for the next forty days and forty nights. If Saint Swithin's Day is dry, the next forty days will also be dry.

WILD HONEYSUCKLE

Keep your eyes open this month for deliciously scented wild honeysuckle twirling its way up trees and hedgerows. Growing honeysuckle around your doorway was believed to bring protection from illness and black magic. Gently crushing fresh flowers on your forehead was said to heighten your psychic powers.

AUGUST

August is another month named after a Roman emperor, this time Augustus, changed from its original name of *"Sextilis"* (being the sixth month in the Roman calendar).

The first of August is Lammas Day and it marks the beginning of the harvest (see page 151).

As well as all the traditional activities surrounding Lammas, it was an opportunity for two young people to enter into a "trial marriage" to see if they were compatible. This marriage usually lasted 11 days and if it didn't work out for them they could separate amicably.

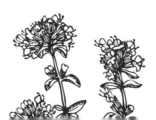
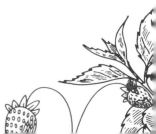

SELF-HEAL

Underneath your feet you may discover this tiny often-overlooked member of the mint family, *Prunella vulgaris*, or "self-heal". Used in a poultice to treat cuts, bruises and bleeding, this herb was so valued as a wound healer that children were told never to pick it or the devil would come in the dead of night and carry them away!

SEPTEMBER

This month's name derives from the Roman word *"septem"*, meaning seven, as September was the seventh month in the Roman calendar.

Michaelmas, also known as the Feast of Saint Michael and All Angels, is celebrated on 29 September every year. In the Middle Ages it was believed that negative forces grew significantly more powerful in the darkness, so with the colder days and darker nights creeping in, Michaelmas marked the beginning of a night curfew. The curfew was signalled by the tolling of the church bell at 9 p.m. every evening, and everyone had to stay safely inside until morning. The bell rang every night until Shrove Tuesday, when the curfew was lifted.

BLACKBERRY

The hedgerows will be fruiting with one of the 330 species of blackberries growing wild in Britain. Taste a few and choose wisely: the sour ones are fine for blackberry vinegar (see page 125), but keep the sweetest of all to enjoy fresh from the bush.

When the devil was thrown out of heaven on Michaelmas Day (29 September) for his proud and arrogant ways, it is said that he fell to Earth and landed on a bramble bush. Cursing the plant for pricking him, he spat on the fruit, turning them sour and making them inedible after this date.

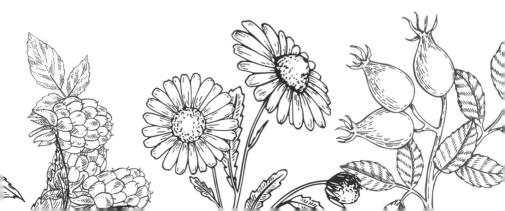

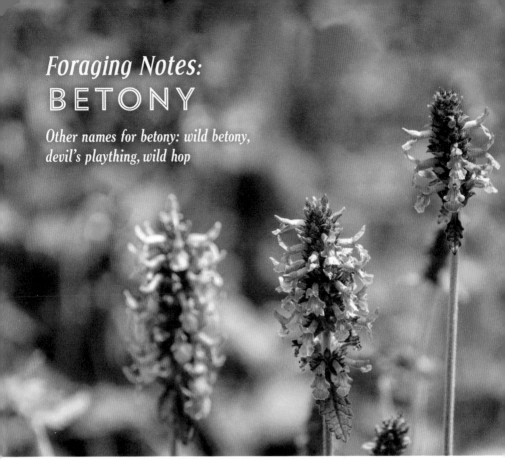

Foraging Notes:
BETONY

Other names for betony: wild betony, devil's plaything, wild hop

HOW TO IDENTIFY: A member of the dead-nettle family, betony's bright magenta pink flowers are almost orchid-like and create striking splashes of colour from early summer well into autumn. Betony can be found growing in light, dry soils on sunny banks and hedgerows or at the edges of ploughed fields. The plant stands up very straight with leaves that are jagged and narrow and mainly found at the base.

COMMON USES: A tea made from betony leaves and flowers is still used by modern herbalists for many complaints such as colds, fevers, poor appetite, sinus trouble and digestive problems.

Betony tea can be prepared by pouring a cup of boiling water on 1 or 2 tsp of the dried leaves and flowers. Allow to stand for 10 to 15 minutes.

Strain and drink, adding a spoonful of honey or agave syrup for sweetness if needed.

NOTES

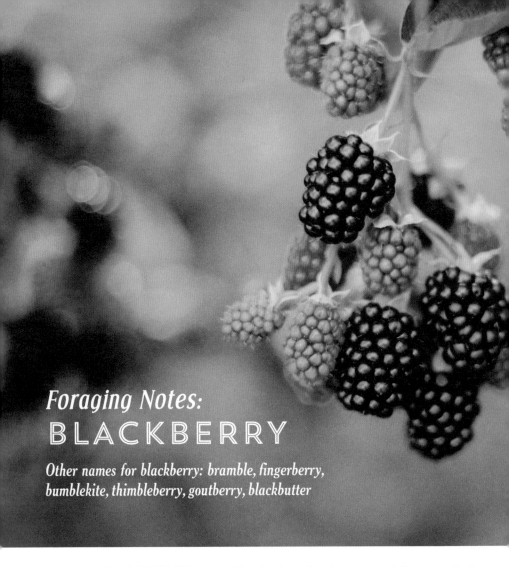

Foraging Notes:
BLACKBERRY

Other names for blackberry: bramble, fingerberry,
bumblekite, thimbleberry, goutberry, blackbutter

HOW TO IDENTIFY: A prickly shrub with white or pink five-petalled flowers, which grows abundantly in the hedgerows and woods from late summer to early autumn. The plump berries turn from green to red to black. The berry at the tip of the thorny stalk is the sweetest of them all, as this is the first to ripen.

COMMON USES: The fruit can be used to make delicious jams, jellies, crumbles and wine. They can also be used to make a slate-blue natural dye, while the roots give an orange colour that can be used to dye wool and cotton.

NOTES

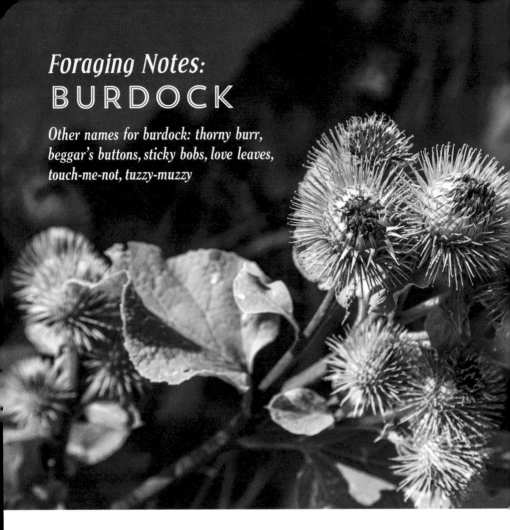

Foraging Notes:
BURDOCK

Other names for burdock: thorny burr,
beggar's buttons, sticky bobs, love leaves,
touch-me-not, tuzzy-muzzy

HOW TO IDENTIFY: A large plant with a long taproot, which is brown or black on the outside. Burdock has outsized, wavy, heart-shaped leaves that are green on the top and whitish underneath and can measure up to 50 cm (20 in.). Purple, thistle-like flowers bloom between June and October, which then turn into hooked seed-bearing burrs that can tangle themselves into animal fur and clothing.

COMMON USES: It is used by modern-day herbalists, who have discovered it to have antibacterial and antifungal properties that are beneficial in the treatment of skin conditions such as eczema. It can also be used to make a lovely dandelion and burdock cordial.

NOTES

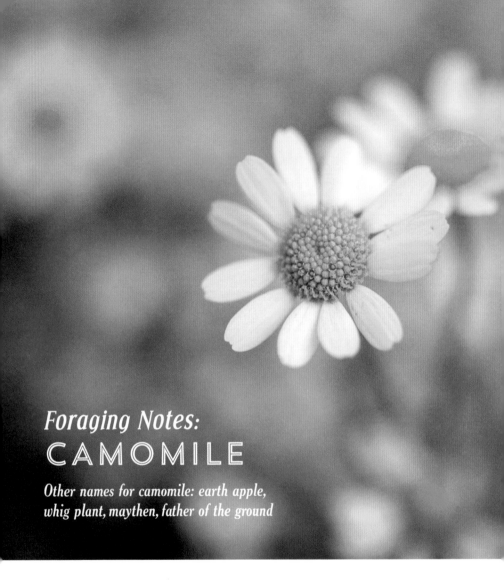

Foraging Notes:
CAMOMILE

*Other names for camomile: earth apple,
whig plant, maythen, father of the ground*

HOW TO IDENTIFY: A small, creeping plant with daisy-like flowers and feathery leaves. One of the best ways to identify camomile is to crush it between your fingers and smell – it should have a pleasant, fresh, apple scent.

COMMON USES: Bunches of camomile plants can be hung in open windows to keep flies away. Camomile infusion makes a lovely rinse to bring out the colour in blonde hair. Of course, camomile tea has long been used to help people relax and get a good night's sleep.

NOTES

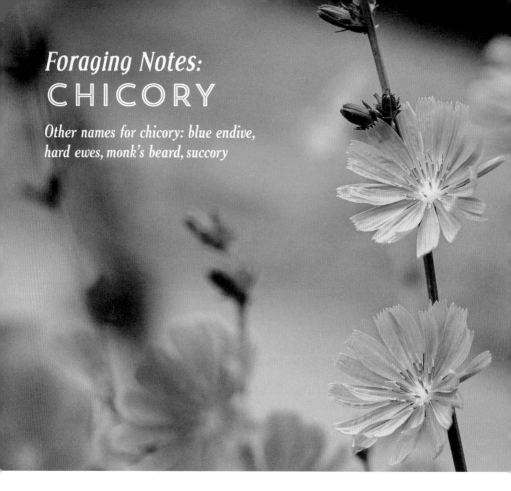

Foraging Notes:
CHICORY

Other names for chicory: blue endive, hard ewes, monk's beard, succory

HOW TO IDENTIFY: The straggly stems of the chicory plant are bedecked with multiple blue daisy-like flowers from July to October. The large-lobed leaves look similar to dandelion leaves with wide gaps that grow smaller toward the tip. Branching stems are covered in fine hairs and have a milky sap inside. Chicory grows in chalky soil and roadside ditches, as well as the disturbed ground at the edge of ploughed fields.

COMMON USES: Chicory leaves can be used to make a blue dye. In the kitchen, chicory leaves can be added to salads and also used as a cooking spice. Chicory root coffee became particularly popular in France in the 1800s when supplies of coffee were scarce due to a trade blockade. Even after coffee became freely available again the French still preferred to blend chicory with their beverage.

NOTES

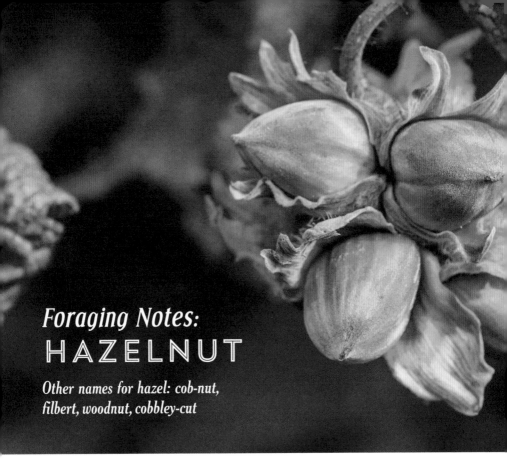

Foraging Notes:
HAZELNUT

Other names for hazel: cob-nut,
filbert, woodnut, cobbley-cut

HOW TO IDENTIFY: Hazel is abundant in the UK. It typically grows to 3–8 m (10–26 ft) tall and can be found in hedgerows and woods. The tooth-edged leaves appear in early May and are often tinged with red, with deep lines running down their length. Flowers appear in autumn and can be open as early as January. The male flower is a long yellow catkin and the female flower is much smaller and bud-like. The female flowers are the ones that develop into delicious hazelnuts, which ripen in late summer and are much coveted by squirrels, mice – and people!

COMMON USES: Woodland crafts using hazel twigs are ever-popular, as the twigs can be twisted and knotted into many shapes. Wild hazelnuts, often called cobnuts, still grow widely in Kent and can be found in native hedgerows – if you can get to them before the squirrels! See page 123 for a recipe for cobnut butter.

NOTES

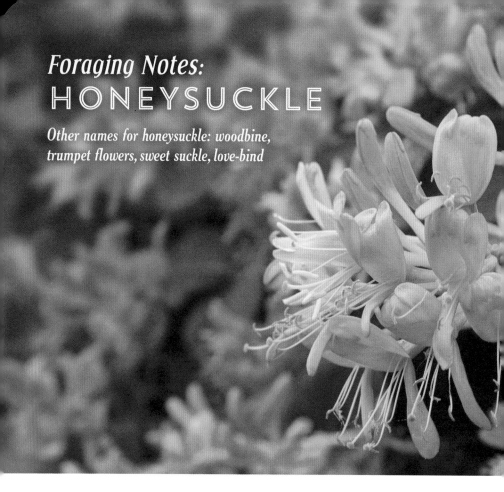

Foraging Notes:
HONEYSUCKLE

Other names for honeysuckle: woodbine, trumpet flowers, sweet suckle, love-bind

HOW TO IDENTIFY: Smaller than the cultivated garden variety, the wild honeysuckle twists and climbs its way up hedgerows and trees, creating a heady, sweet scent that is carried on the breeze. Distinctive yellowy-white, trumpet-like flowers appear in summer, attracting pollinators at dusk when their scent is at its most fragrant. Clusters of red berries ripen in the autumn to be gratefully devoured by warblers, thrushes and bullfinches, but they are sadly not safe for human consumption.

COMMON USES: The flowers can be used in teas, jellies and jams, for making country wine and for decorating cakes. Pour raw honey over honeysuckle flowers in a jam jar until they are completely covered, pop on the lid and place in a cool dark place for four weeks. Remove the flowers and keep the honey to use as a remedy to ease sore throats and coughs.

NOTES

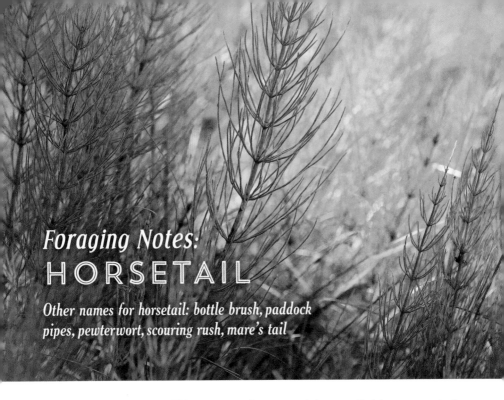

Foraging Notes:
HORSETAIL

Other names for horsetail: bottle brush, paddock pipes, pewterwort, scouring rush, mare's tail

HOW TO IDENTIFY: Deep in the ground, horsetail rhizomes wait for spring before showing their parasol-shaped stems above ground. Commonly found on waste ground, railway embankments and fields, the plants grow to around 80 cm (30 in.) tall. They do not have hairs or leaves but bristles, formed by thin, barren stems. Horsetail doesn't flower; it reproduces in the same way as ferns, with spores that are produced in the cone-shaped clusters of small green branches. These tufty green branches produce quite a haze of green foliage and the plant closely resembles a bottle brush.

COMMON USES: In modern herbal medicine, horsetail is used for fluid retention, kidney and bladder stones and urine infections, as well as osteoporosis. It can improve brittle fingernails and help with the production of collagen for healthy skin and shiny hair. You can also make a healthy hair mist by infusing boiled spring water with dried horsetail and nettle leaves and mixing in aloe vera and rosemary, lavender and clary sage essential oils (shake well before each use). Soaking your fingernails in an infusion of chopped horsetail can help to strengthen brittle nails – make sure you do it several times a week to get the full benefit.

NOTES

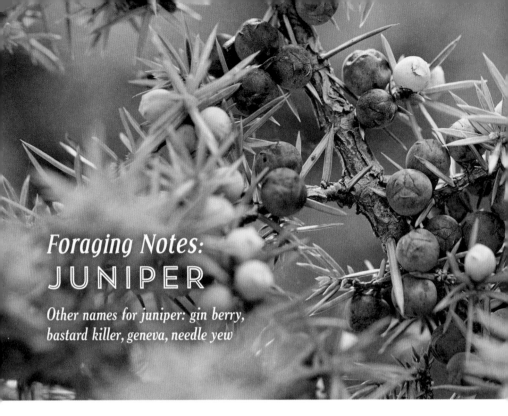

Foraging Notes:
JUNIPER

Other names for juniper: gin berry,
bastard killer, geneva, needle yew

HOW TO IDENTIFY: Juniper is one of the characteristic heathland shrubs of chalk and limestone areas. The leaves take the form of needles and are a deep green colour, sometimes with a bluish tinge. On account of its needle-like leaves, it is often known in folk tradition as the "needle yew". The berries usually take two to three years to ripen fully; it is common to see both the bluish-black ripe berries alongside very green and under-ripe ones on the same bush. When fully ripe, the berries are about the size of a pea and have an aromatic, resiny scent.

COMMON USES: Juniper berries are still widely used in French and southern European recipes as a complement to venison, mutton or lamb. It's best not to eat them raw as they can cause stomach upsets. Juniper oil is used in the perfume industry for its masculine scent. Alternatively, you can use the berries to create a warming foot bath to revive your feet after a long day's foraging – just tie berries, cloves, rosehips, orange peel and dried hibiscus in a muslin bag and infuse in boiling water, then add cold water until it's a bearable temperature to soak your feet.

NOTES

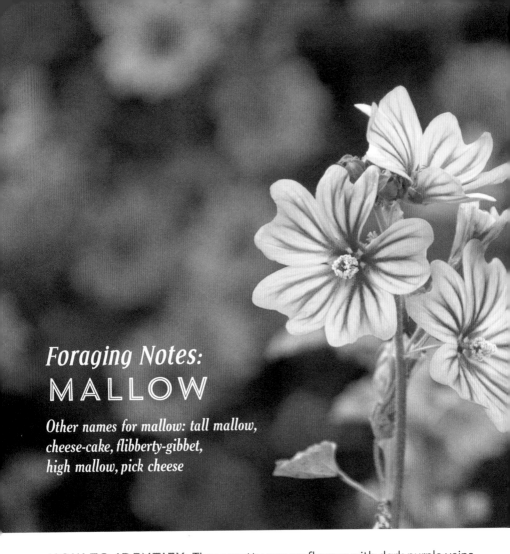

Foraging Notes:
MALLOW

Other names for mallow: tall mallow, cheese-cake, flibberty-gibbet, high mallow, pick cheese

HOW TO IDENTIFY: These pretty mauve flowers with dark purple veins appear from June to September in sheltered, well-drained places. The ivy-shaped leaves have five to seven lobes with a covering of downy hair. The fruit are commonly called "cheeses" because they closely resemble truckles of cheese.

COMMON USES: Marshmallow is still used today in the treatment of coughs and sore throats, (some cough sweets contain mallow). It is also used as a laxative, so don't overindulge! Marshmallow leaf and root can be applied as a poultice for insect bites, skin inflammation or minor burns.

NOTES

Foraging Notes:
MEADOWSWEET

Other names for meadowsweet:
bridewort, lady of the meadow,
summer's farewell, old man's pepper

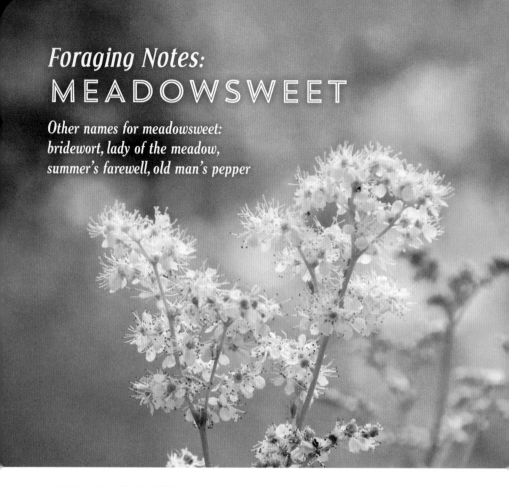

HOW TO IDENTIFY: Meadowsweet dwells on riverbanks and in damp meadows and ditches. It flowers from June to September and is identifiable by its frothy clusters of upright, sweet-smelling, clotted-cream-coloured flowers, which have an attractive vanilla/almond scent. The red stems grow to about 1.5 m (5 ft) tall and, surprisingly, it is a member of the rose family, as shown by the shape of its red-tinged leaves.

COMMON USES: Meadowsweet flowers can be used to flavour wines, vinegars, beer, claret and a delicious cordial. For meadowsweet syrup, strip the flowers from their stalks, place them in a cafetière and fill with boiling water. Push the plunger down and leave for 2 hours, then strain. For every 100 ml of liquid stir in 50 ml honey or maple syrup. Keep in a sterilized bottle in the fridge and use (topped up with sparkling water) within a week.

NOTES

Foraging Notes:
MUGWORT

*Other names for mugwort:
maiden's wort, naughty man, crone
wort, witch herb, sailor's tobacco*

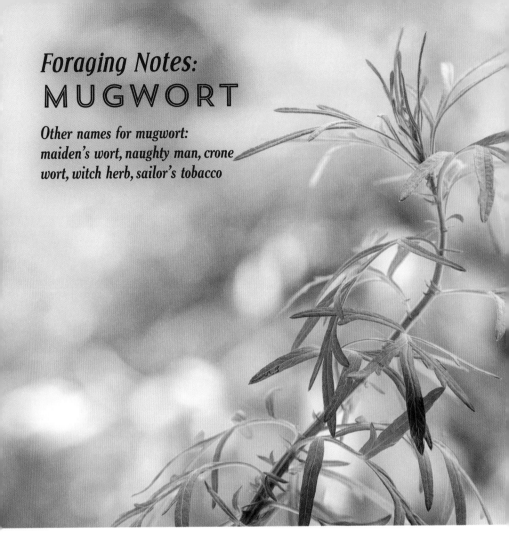

HOW TO IDENTIFY: This hardy plant grows on wasteland and verges and it can grow up to 2 m (6½ ft) tall. The leaves are delicate and finely lobed, dark green on the uppermost side and covered in dense silvery hairs on the underside. Mugwort is in bloom from June to September, with tiny clusters of whitish-green flowers and a distinct fragrance of sage.

COMMON USES: An infusion of mugwort leaves can be used as an environmentally friendly plant spray to repel insects. Use with care as it can also inhibit plant growth if overused.

Dried mugwort can be hung in a wardrobe to deter moths.

NOTES

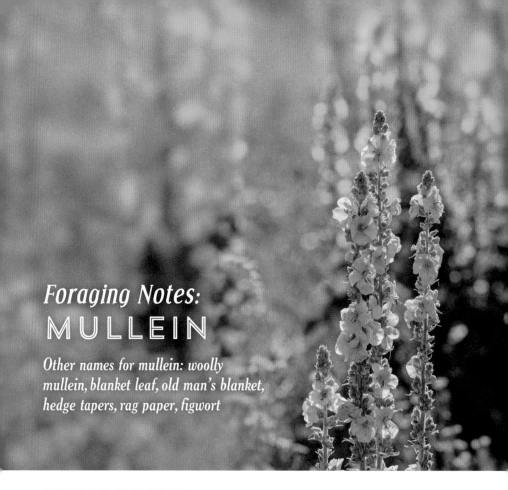

Foraging Notes:
MULLEIN

*Other names for mullein: woolly
mullein, blanket leaf, old man's blanket,
hedge tapers, rag paper, figwort*

HOW TO IDENTIFY: The distinctive flower spikes of the mullein grow to over 2 m (6½ ft) tall and can be found on railway embankments, open fields or anywhere that is dry and sunny. The silvery leaves have soft hairs with the feel of thick felt – no surprise, then, that they have often been used as nature's toilet paper for people caught short in the countryside! Pale yellow, saucer-shaped flowers climb around the flower spike and are in bloom throughout summer.

COMMON USES: To remove splinters and draw out boils, lay a mullein leaf in a dish, pour over a little boiling water and leave to cool. Wrap around the affected part and secure with a bandage. The leaves and flowers can be used to make tea to help relieve coughs and chesty colds. Mullein flowers and garlic infused into olive oil can be used as eardrops to help ease earache.

NOTES

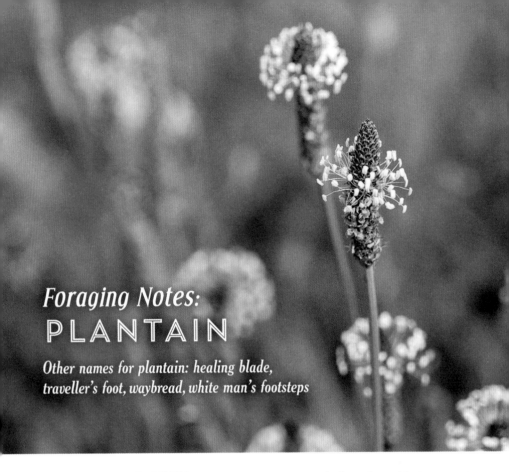

Foraging Notes:
PLANTAIN

Other names for plantain: healing blade,
traveller's foot, waybread, white man's footsteps

HOW TO IDENTIFY: A ubiquitous perennial plant found in lawns, at roadsides and on footpaths (not to be mistaken for the Caribbean banana variety). Described by some as a short, fat, ugly weed, the plantain is actually one of the best healing herbs.

The broad, oval-shaped leaves grow in a rosette with distinctive stringy veins running from the bottom to the top. The long, slender flower stalks grow from the central core, with many tiny greenish-yellow flowers that produce hundreds of seeds.

COMMON USES: Young leaves can be put in salads, although they can be rather bitter. The leaves, which are antibacterial and anti-inflammatory, are a traditional remedy for insect or nettle stings. Chew the leaves before using on the skin as the enzymes in saliva help to release the active constituents needed for healing.

NOTES

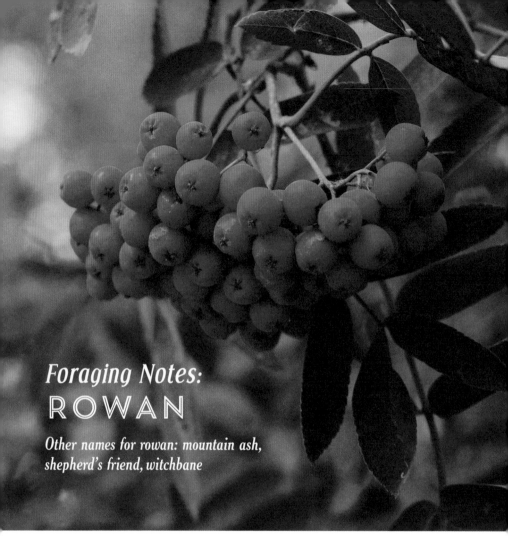

Foraging Notes:
ROWAN

Other names for rowan: mountain ash, shepherd's friend, witchbane

HOW TO IDENTIFY: The rowan is a small, grey-barked tree that is common in rocky places and dry, wooded areas. The leaves are feather-like, comprising five to eight pairs of distinctive serrated leaflets.

The flower heads, which appear from May to June, are buttery white with five petals on flat branched clusters. In autumn, the leaves turn a brilliant flame colour, dangling with round, fleshy, scarlet fruits.

COMMON USES: Rowan berries were successfully used to treat scurvy as they are rich in vitamins A and C. The berries ripen in October and are tastiest when cooked with other fruits to make jams and jellies.

NOTES

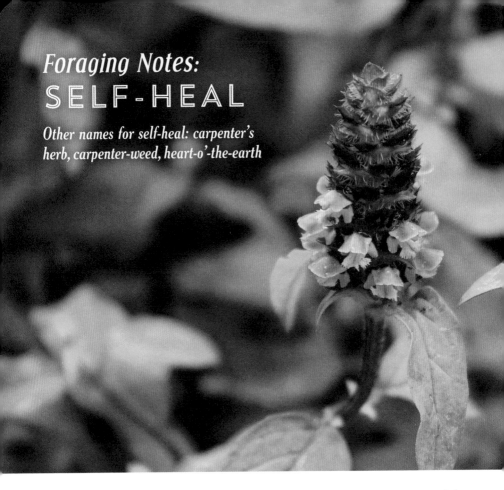

Foraging Notes:
SELF-HEAL

Other names for self-heal: carpenter's herb, carpenter-weed, heart-o'-the-earth

HOW TO IDENTIFY: This low-growing perennial herb is a member of the mint family and can be seen creeping along roadside verges and popping up in untreated lawns. Clusters of small, lip-shaped purple flowers appear on top of square-stemmed spikes from June through to early autumn. It loves damp shady places and is a very important source of nectar for bees and wasps.

COMMON USES: Through a series of modern clinical trials and studies, self-heal has been found to have powerful antiviral properties that combat coughs, colds and fever symptoms. It is effective against a range of bacteria including the one that causes tuberculosis. Infuse the dried leaves and flowers into 100 ml of carrier oil by warming it gently in a heatproof bowl over a pan of boiling water for 1 hour. Stir in 15 g of beeswax and then pour into sterilized jars for a simple remedy for prickly heat or nettle rash.

NOTES

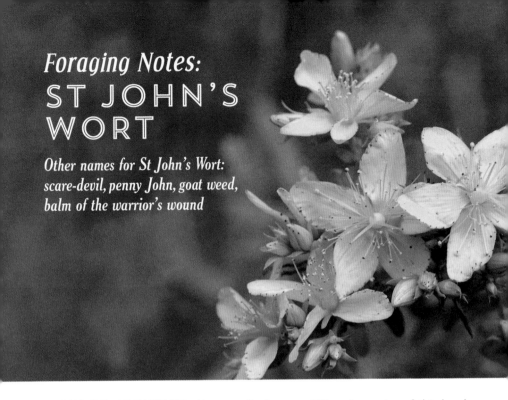

Foraging Notes:
ST JOHN'S WORT

Other names for St John's Wort:
scare-devil, penny John, goat weed,
balm of the warrior's wound

HOW TO IDENTIFY: You can find many different species of this lovely plant along the June hedgerow. The bright yellow, star-shaped flowers bloom all summer long. The leaves are easily recognizable as they are about 1.5 cm (½ in.) long and have a perforated appearance: these are actually oil glands, not holes. It grows to about 1 m (3 ft) tall and readily self-seeds.

This plant blooms during the summer solstice and is believed to be at its most powerful when the sun is at its peak on 24 June, which is St John's Day.

COMMON USES: The fresh flowers and buds of St John's Wort are used by herbalists as a treatment for seasonal affective disorder (SAD) and the darkness of depression. It is also used to ease the discomfort of shingles as it is antiviral and has pain-relieving qualities, too. You can make your own healing salve by putting the flowering tops in a jar and covering with a carrier oil (almond or olive work well) and leaving on a sunny windowsill for a month. Be careful, though, as the oil could make your skin more sensitive to the sun.

*This herb should not be taken internally without the advice of a qualified herbalist.

NOTES

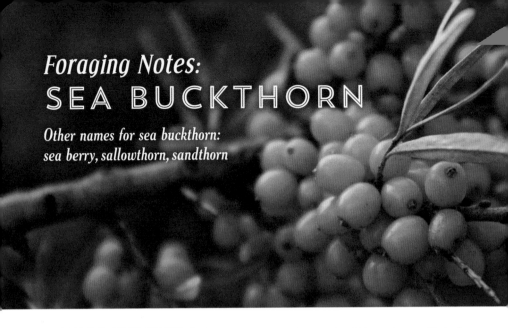

Foraging Notes:
SEA BUCKTHORN

Other names for sea buckthorn:
sea berry, sallowthorn, sandthorn

HOW TO IDENTIFY: As its name suggests, sea buckthorn is mostly to be found in coastal areas, especially around sand dunes where it helps to stabilize the soil, and is also often planted along roadsides. Growing to about 2.5 m (8 ft) tall with long thin greyish green leaves, it forms dense thickets with thorny twigs. The distinctive bright orange berries provide tasty food for thrushes as they arrive from the continent.

The plant is covered in unfriendly spikes and the berries burst very easily when you try to pick them. However, as it's only really the juice that you're after, you can take a plastic container along with you and some gloves and just squeeze some juice from the berries into your container while they're still on the bush.

Folklore tells us that sea buckthorn leaves were the favourite food of the mythical flying horse Pegasus. The ancient Greeks also fed the leaves to their ailing or injured horses to make them healthy and strong again; the Latin name for sea buckthorn is *"Hippophae"* meaning "shining horse".

COMMON USES: The bright orange berries literally burst with vitamin C and antioxidants, making it a great remedy for winter ailments – although you may have to sweeten the raw juice considerably to make it palatable. Simply pour your sea buckthorn juice through a sieve, squashing the flesh to extract the maximum amount of liquid, whisk in runny honey or maple syrup to taste and dilute with still or sparkling water.

NOTES

OTHER
FORAGING FINDS

WILD STRAWBERRY

Look carefully on open woodland, grassy banks of chalk downland and limestone and you may be lucky enough to be rewarded with tasty little wild strawberries. This beauty, which is not actually related to the cultivated strawberry that we now know, was being foraged by our ancestors in the Stone Age. Wild strawberry plants grow to about 30 cm (12 in.) with trefoil leaves and white flowers giving way to tiny scarlet fruit in early summer. Due to their small size it's unlikely that you'll be able to forage enough wild strawberries to make into jam, so enjoy them instead as a sweet treat while you walk. Remember to leave some for the wildlife to enjoy, too.

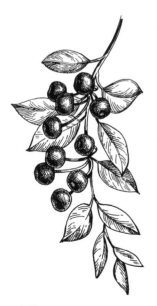

WILD CHERRY

If you happen upon a tree full of ripe wild cherries, pick a few as soon as you can before native birds make short work of them. The cherry is a tall tree that can reach up to 5 m (16 ft) in height, with masses of snowy white or pink blossom in the spring, followed by delicious red fleshy fruits in early summer. Wild cherries are often smaller than cultivated ones and tend to be sharper-tasting, so are best used in recipes involving sugar or honey.

FAT HEN

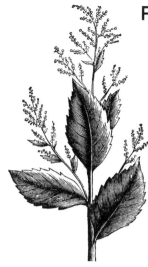

Another plant that would have been included in our ancestors' everlasting pottage pot, fat hen can be discovered growing in disturbed ground, wasteland, along roadsides and round the edges of farmers' fields – try to look for areas with weeds, as these spots are less likely to have been sprayed with pesticides. Dull diamond-shaped leaves with a silvery sheen make it look very similar to spinach. The leaves, which are a good source of vitamins and minerals, can be eaten raw in salad or cooked in the same way as spinach, and the tiny white flowers are edible, too.

WALNUTS

The common English walnut was first introduced to our countryside by the Romans. Today they can be found in hedgerows, woodlands and wasteland, and have been known to grow to 50 m (164 ft) in height. You'll notice bright green tennis-ball-sized globes beginning to fall to the ground in late summer. Wear gloves to break them open as they can stain your skin. Inside is the familiar brown walnut shell – allow these to dry out for a few days then crack them open and enjoy.

Walnut shells have long been used to make dye for natural fibres, with colours ranging from beige to dark brown. To 25 g of walnut shells add 250 ml of boiling water in a saucepan, and simmer with the lid on for 8 hours, or until reduced by about half. For an even darker ink add a few rusty nails to the pan. Add ½ tsp of both vinegar and salt and stir to dissolve. Carefully strain the liquid and pour into a glass jar and seal tightly.

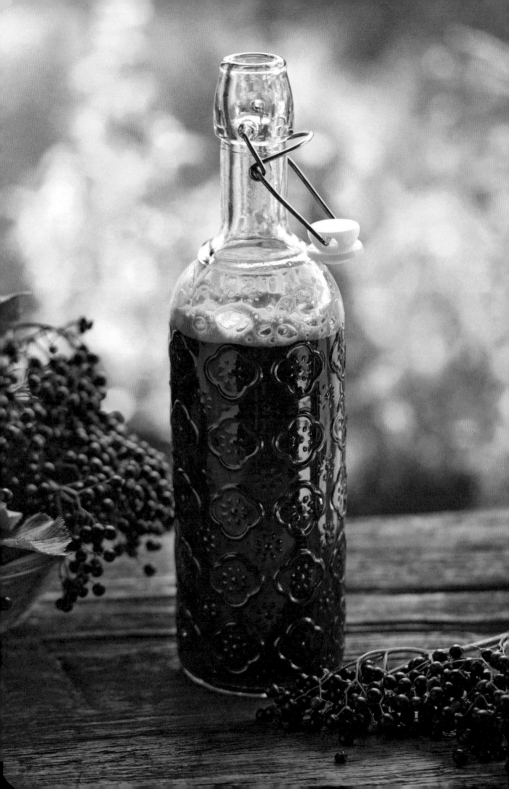

ELDERBERRY ROB

Elderberries have wonderful antiviral and antioxidant properties, so it's worth freezing some so you can whip up a batch of this medicinal rob any time of year to speed up recovery from coughs, colds and sore throats. The addition of cloves not only helps to preserve the rob but also lends it their own antiviral and antibacterial benefits. Heat it up for an extra-soothing drink, or add a little rum or brandy and a squeeze of lemon for a medicinal hot toddy.

Be fussy when you pick elderberries as shrivelled berries won't give up much juice.

Makes around 750 ml

INGREDIENTS

500 g ripe elderberries – either fresh or frozen – you can leave them on the stalk

Water

10–15 whole cloves, approximately

300–450 g caster sugar, approximately

Sterilized bottles

METHOD

Place your berries in a large pan. Ensure it is large enough not to boil over. Add water until the berries are just floating.

Slowly bring to the boil and simmer for 15 minutes.

Use a potato masher to burst any berries that are still whole.

Carefully pour the liquid through a colander and into a large jug, using the masher to squeeze out as much juice as you can. It's worth taking time to do this as the best juice comes out right at the end.

Pour the liquid through a sieve and measure your juice into a pan. For every 500 ml of juice, add 300 g of sugar and ten cloves.

Bring slowly to the boil, stirring constantly to dissolve the sugar. Bring to a rolling boil for 5 minutes, then allow to cool slightly before pouring into sterile bottles and labelling.

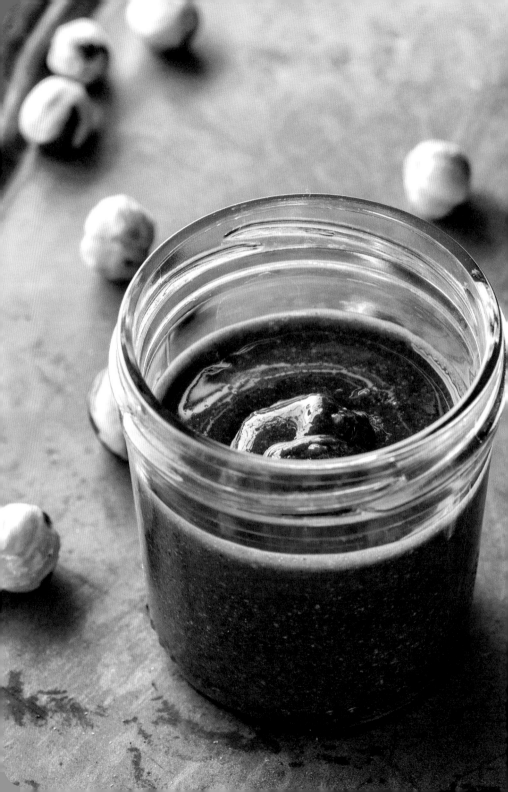

HAZELNUT BUTTER

I just love making nut butters! They taste great, are free from the palm oil often included in commercial nut butters, and are rich in magnesium, calcium, unsaturated fats and vitamins B and E. Plus, they are delicious and really easy to make!

Makes approximately one 500-g jar

INGREDIENTS

400 g blanched hazelnuts or cobnuts

3 tbsp organic cacao powder

2 tbsp maple syrup

½ tsp sea salt

METHOD

Roast your hazelnuts on a baking tray at 180°C (356°F) for about ten minutes or until golden brown. They burn easily, so keep watch! Allow to cool.

Tip the nuts into a food processor, add the cacao, maple syrup and salt. It is possible to blend them with a pestle and mortar, but it will be very hard work!

Grind for about five minutes, stopping to push the mixture down occasionally. At first it will just look like sand, but be patient...

And, as if by magic, it will suddenly turn into a creamy, velvety butter. Keep whizzing until it is completely smooth.

If you feel it is too thick, add a drizzle of hazelnut or sunflower oil and grind again.

Spoon into a clean, dry jar.

The same recipe works just as well using peanuts.

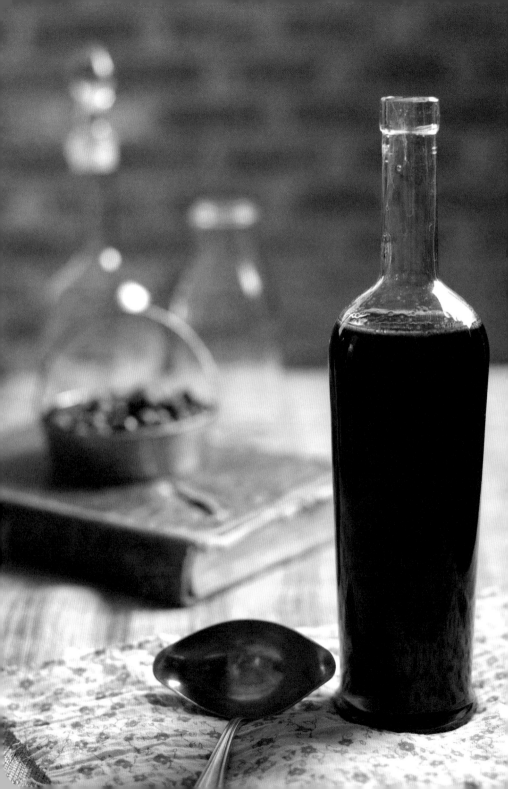

WILD BLACKBERRY VINEGAR

Blackberries are an excellent source of the powerful antioxidant vitamins A, C and K. At the first sign of a prickly sore throat, gargle with a spoonful of this vinegar to ease symptoms. It also makes a delicious salad dressing when mixed with an oil of your choice, or use two teaspoons when making meringues to give a chewy texture. Collect your blackberries on a dry day, from a hedgerow away from busy roads.

Makes approximately 500 ml

INGREDIENTS

300 g blackberries

300 g caster sugar

300 ml white wine vinegar

METHOD

Rinse your blackberries in cold water and pat dry with a clean tea towel, allowing any little bugs to escape. Put the berries into a large jar or bowl and cover with white wine vinegar until they are just floating. Cover and place somewhere cool for five to seven days, stirring every day to release the lovely purple colour.

At the end of that time, strain the vinegar from the berries through a fine sieve into a jug. Allow the liquid to drip through overnight.

Measure the vinegar and pour it into a large saucepan. For every 100 ml of vinegar, add 50 g of caster sugar. Slowly bring to the boil, stirring constantly to dissolve the sugar, then bring to a rolling boil for 5 minutes.

Allow the liquid to cool for 10 minutes, pour into sterilized bottles, cap tightly and label.

Use within one year.

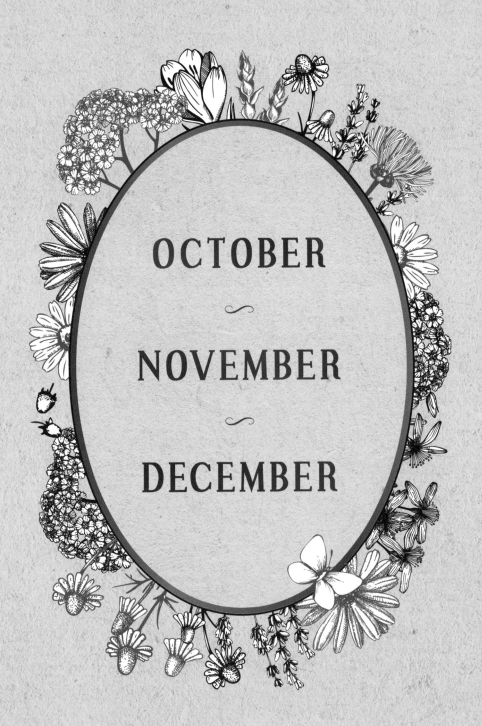

OCTOBER

∽

NOVEMBER

∽

DECEMBER

Without a doubt autumn is my favourite season: the nights are getting longer, the days shorter and there is the promise of winter in the air. Harvest festival is being celebrated in every church up and down the country, the fruit trees are ready and squashes, pumpkins and root vegetables are plentiful.

John Keats paints a beautiful picture of the bounty available at this time of year in his poem, "To Autumn": "To bend with apples the moss'd cottage trees. And fill all fruit with ripeness to the core. To swell the gourd, and plump the hazel shells with sweet kernel."

Autumn was a very busy time for our ancestors, who would still be storing fruit, salting meat and gathering in the last of the grain harvest, as well as ensuring that they had enough wood to keep the fire going for cooking throughout the winter. Straw was dried thoroughly for animal bedding and winter fodder. Grain lasted well but had to be kept safely away from rats, mice and other vermin. Autumn was the season of careful preparation; harvesting and storing sufficient food for the winter really was a matter of life and death.

One of the plants that comes into its own at this time of year is the rose plant, whose rosehips shine out of the hedgerows like fairy lights. It's well worth braving their unforgiving thorns to gather some for syrups and jellies, but always remove the itchy hairs inside for safety (as these can irritate mucous membranes).

The holy grail of the autumn hedgerows has to be the umbrella-shaped dark purple clusters of drooping elderberries; our native birds enjoy them, too, and it's advisable to pick them immediately, otherwise the birds will strip every single berry.

Beware: there are some elderberry look-a-likes in the hedgerow, so when in doubt, leave it out! Respect nature and don't be tempted to pick more than you really need, as the birds and squirrels rely heavily on autumn fruit to see them through the lean winter months.

Crab apple fruit is easily identified, and although too bitter to eat raw, it makes great crab apple jelly. Purple-black sloes should be picked when the fruit gives slightly when squeezed, and they will make sloe gin in time for Christmas.

Avoid foraging in the rain as excess moisture will cause your fruits to grow mildew, especially if you carry them home in a plastic bag – wicker baskets prevent bruising and allow the fruit to breathe, keeping it fresher for longer.

WHERE TO GO

In the autumn, leaves are turning from green to red to gold, there's a nip in the air and the hedgerows and woodlands are full of nuts and berries waiting to be foraged from the countryside and urban spaces. Elderberries, sloes and rosehips adorn the hedgerows, sweet chestnuts are falling from the trees and there is still sheep's sorrel and nettles to be gathered in your local park or on the woodland floor. Keep your eyes on the ground for the many varieties of fungi that will also be making an appearance – take photographs, but don't forage mushrooms unless you are with a qualified expert.

FOLKLORE AND TRADITIONS

OCTOBER

October was originally the eighth month in the Julian calendar (*"Octo"* meaning "eight" in Latin). October was traditionally the time for "mop" fairs – otherwise known as "hiring" fairs – when anyone looking for work would make themselves available to potential employers. They would attend mop fairs dressed in their Sunday best and carrying something that signified their trade – a mop for a maid, vegetables or flowers for a gardener and wool for a shepherd.

DOG ROSE

Bright red rosehips will appear on the dog rose in the hedgerows about now. Folklore tells us that if you carry one in your pocket it will prevent you from getting piles. Faeries who wish to become invisible will eat a rosehip and turn three times widdershins (anti-clockwise). To reappear, they eat another rosehip and turn three times sunwise (clockwise).

NOVEMBER

November comes from the Latin word *"novem"*, meaning "nine". Our medieval ancestors celebrated the feast of Martinmas on 11 November, marking the end of the farming year with the successful planting of the wheat. A great feast was prepared for all farm workers and their families, where goose was the traditional food, fires were lit and children carried lanterns. The goose was a particularly important part of the feast as it was believed that the markings on the breast bones of the bird could predict the severity of the coming winter and whether it would come early or late in the year.

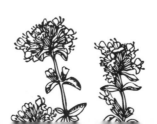
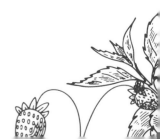

BLACKTHORN

Early November is the time to gather sloes from the blackthorn tree in order to make sloe gin for Christmas.

Devon witches were said to carry walking sticks made from blackthorn wood and also to use the nasty sharp thorns to pierce effigies called "poppets", which were made in the image of an enemy.

DECEMBER

Another month that retained its original name, from *"decem"*, meaning "ten", despite being moved to the twelfth month with the adoption of the Gregorian calendar.

On Boxing Day rich employers would give their servants a "Christmas Box" of money to show their gratitude for their hard work in the previous year. This courtesy was often extended to reliable tradespeople such as grocers and bakers to ensure good service and the best goods for the following year.

PINE

If you have an open fire at home you can dry out foraged pinecones and use them as natural firelighters – dip them into melted candle wax to make them even more efficient. Pine cones were said to represent spiritual enlightenment, which is why you will see pine cones used in some Catholic symbolism and also on top of some ecclesiastical lanterns and candle holders.

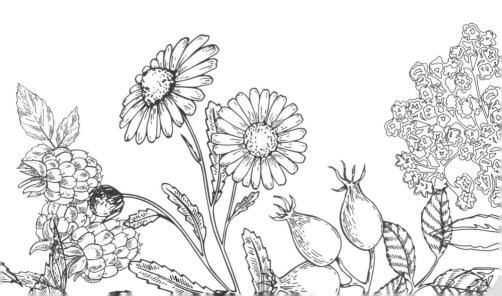

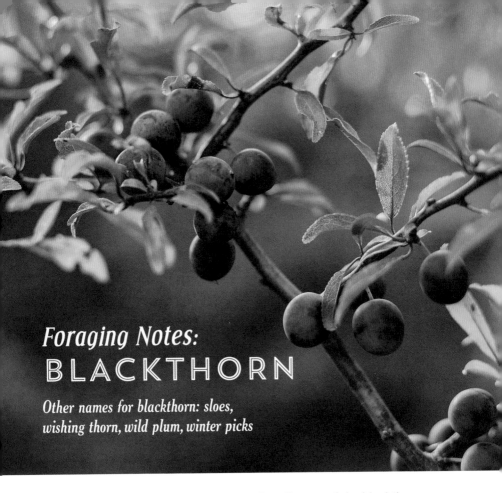

Foraging Notes:
BLACKTHORN

Other names for blackthorn: sloes,
wishing thorn, wild plum, winter picks

HOW TO IDENTIFY: The snowy white flowers of the blackthorn are one of the first blooms of spring in the hedgerow. The blackthorn can grow to over 3 m (10 ft) tall. It has thorny branches, small oval-shaped leaves and purple marble-sized fruits, commonly known as sloes.

COMMON USES: The best use of sloes by far is sloe gin! Put 500 g sloes and 250 g caster sugar into a sterilized 1 litre jar and pour over 70 cl of gin. Shake well to dissolve the sugar.

Store the jar in a dark cupboard for at least two months, remembering to shake the jar occasionally. Sieve out the fruit and decant the liquor into clean bottles.

Don't throw away your sloes after you've made your sloe gin – use them to make delicious sloe port (see page 147).

NOTES

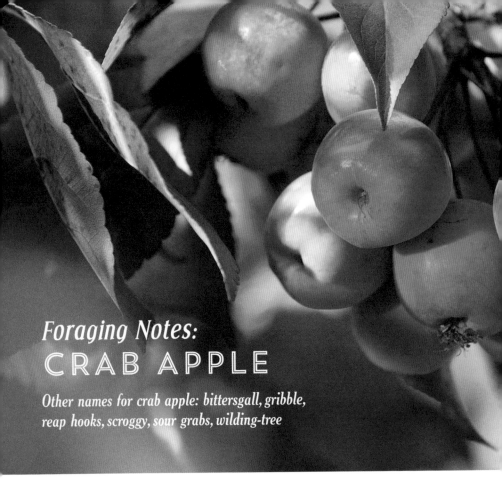

Foraging Notes:
CRAB APPLE

Other names for crab apple: bittersgall, gribble, reap hooks, scroggy, sour grabs, wilding-tree

HOW TO IDENTIFY: This wild native species is a diminutive thorny tree that can be found in woodland edges and hedgerows. The deciduous leaves are arranged alternately on the branches and can vary in shape but are roughly oval or round, with a pointed end and finely serrated edges. As the tree grows older the scaly, greyish bark becomes cracked, twisted and gnarly. The five-petalled pink flowers bloom in the hedgerow in spring, usually between April and May. Crab apples are sharper and smaller than cultivated apples and may be green, yellow or red in colour. The stalk is long in relation to the size of the fruit when compared to a standard-size common apple.

COMMON USES: Their bitter, dry taste makes them unpalatable when raw, but their intense apple flavour works well in many recipes, including drinks and jams. Crab apples are also used as a pollinator for other fruits.

NOTES

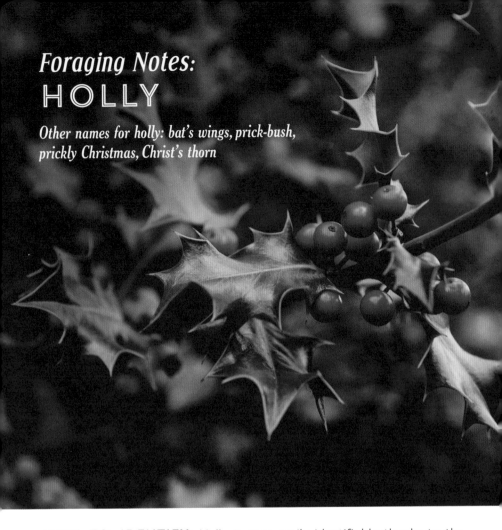

Foraging Notes:
HOLLY

Other names for holly: bat's wings, prick-bush, prickly Christmas, Christ's thorn

HOW TO IDENTIFY: Holly is very easily identifiable thanks to the popularity of holly wreaths and holly images on Christmas cards. This evergreen shrub can grow to 15 m (50 ft) tall and live for 200 years or more. Leaves are glossy, thick, dark green and usually prickly; they grow alternately on the stems. Once pollinated by insects, the white female flowers are followed by the familiar red or orange berries that remain on the tree throughout winter.

COMMON USES: Holly hedges and trees provide vital food and shelter for our native birds through winter and a lovely addition to our natural decorations for the festive season.

NOTES

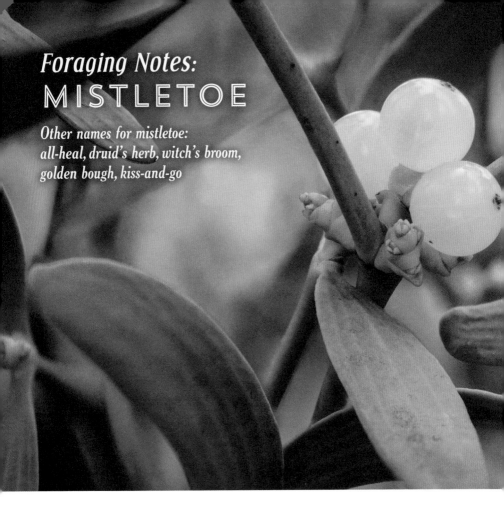

Foraging Notes:
MISTLETOE

Other names for mistletoe:
all-heal, druid's herb, witch's broom,
golden bough, kiss-and-go

HOW TO IDENTIFY: This parasitic plant with its globe-like form is easy to spot on the bare branches of winter trees. Mistletoe is the only plant to have all three of these distinctive features – forked branches, pearlescent white berries and evergreen pairs of elongated oval leaves. It most commonly grows on apple, lime and hawthorn trees.

All parts are poisonous to animals and it is not recommended for human consumption unless prescribed by a medical herbalist. Wear gloves to avoid contact.

COMMON USES: Christmas wouldn't be Christmas without a sprig of mistletoe hanging in the doorway, or use it in your festive door wreath to symbolize hospitality and peace within.

NOTES

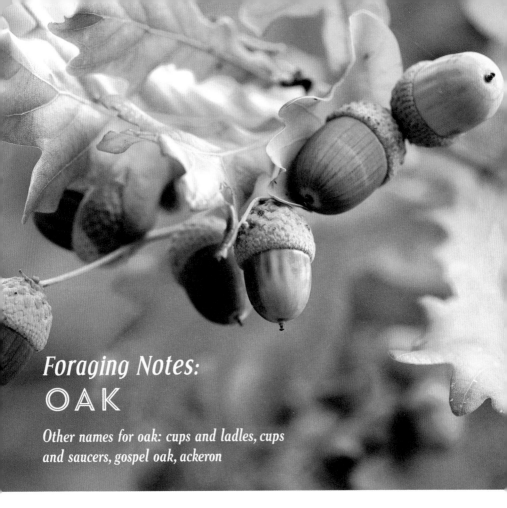

Foraging Notes:
OAK

Other names for oak: cups and ladles, cups and saucers, gospel oak, ackeron

HOW TO IDENTIFY: This much-admired deciduous tree can grow to well over 30 m (about 100 ft) tall. It has a broad-spreading crown that allows light to fall on the woodland floor below.

The lobed leaves burst into life in bunches around May, followed by long yellow catkins that blow in the breeze, distributing their pollen. Acorn fruits follow the catkins, which ripen to a nutty brown and fall to the ground in the autumn when they are gathered by hungry squirrels and other hedgerow dwellers.

COMMON USES: Surprisingly, many things can be made from acorns, from coffee substitutes to acorn flour. They can also be useful in art and craft projects to decorate homemade wreaths, and acorn cups make the most delightful floating faerie candles.

NOTES

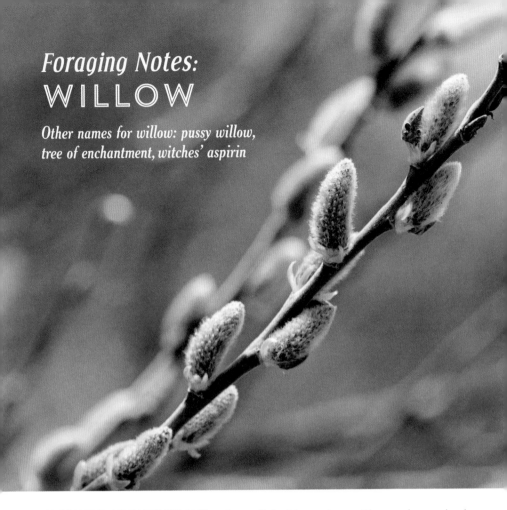

Foraging Notes:
WILLOW

*Other names for willow: pussy willow,
tree of enchantment, witches' aspirin*

HOW TO IDENTIFY: Willow is a tall deciduous tree with grey-brown bark that develops deep cracks over time. Willow can be found along riverbanks, in wet woodlands and around lakes. Long yellow catkins appear in spring, providing much-needed nectar for insects that, in return, pollinate the tree. The slender, oval-shaped leaves are covered on the underside with silky hairs, which make them appear white as the wind tumbles them.

COMMON USES: The twigs are long, slender and very flexible, making them useful for various crafts. Some of the many uses for willow include: wicker baskets, willow screens, shelters and sculptures, woven fences and willow wreaths. Willow can also be made into drawing charcoal, which has been used by artists for centuries.

NOTES

OTHER FORAGING FINDS

SWEET CHESTNUT

Belonging to the same family as oak and beech, this giant of a tree can grow up to 35 m (115 ft) tall and is found in woodlands particularly in the south-east of Britain. The shiny brown edible sweet chestnuts are wrapped in a very spiky bright green casing which can be found littering the forest floor in the autumn. Don't confuse them with conkers from the horse chestnut tree, which have a brown casing and are toxic and are definitely not for eating.

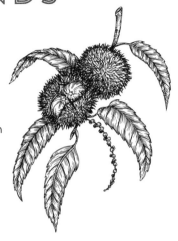

In folklore sweet chestnuts are eaten as an aphrodisiac and carried around by women who wish to improve their chances of conceiving.

Chestnuts have a rich, nutty flavour and can be gathered now to keep for roasting at Christmas, used in stuffing or ground into flour for baking and as a thickener for soup and gravy.

HORSERADISH

You can find this fiery plant (most commonly used for the popular condiment) growing in areas that have previously been disturbed, such as farmland, grass verges and along roadsides. The leaves grow tall and are shiny with a wavy edge, and they emit their distinct smell when you crush them – a good way of distinguishing them from dock, which looks quite similar. Horseradish was originally only considered to be fit for farm labourers and poor people to eat in the Middle Ages, but by the seventeenth century it was being eaten with beef and oysters by all classes of Englishman, as well as being made into a spicy cordial to revive weary travellers.

Young horseradish leaves can be eaten raw or cooked, but now is the time to harvest the root to turn into horseradish sauce. The roots go down very deep so you may need a shovel or fork to get at them. Always ask the landowner's permission before you dig up any root.

DAMSONS

Finding a damson tree heaving with fruit is a joy indeed. A member of the plum family, damsons are small, oval fruits (similar to regular plums) that are deep purple in colour, with a bluish bloom over the skin similar to sloes. They have a fruity tartness that is much sourer than plums. The leaves are dark green and shiny with a serrated edge. Damson trees grow in woodlands and can also be found in hedgerows, gardens and parks. Damson trees don't tend to grow overly tall, meaning the fruit is easier to pick.

Damson jam is one of my absolute favourite things to make with these sour fruits, but you can also substitute them for sloes to make damson gin or vodka, or cook them up in a crumble – you may need to add quite a lot of sugar to combat the sourness, though!

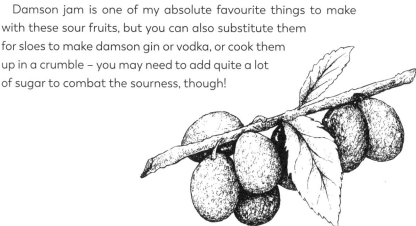

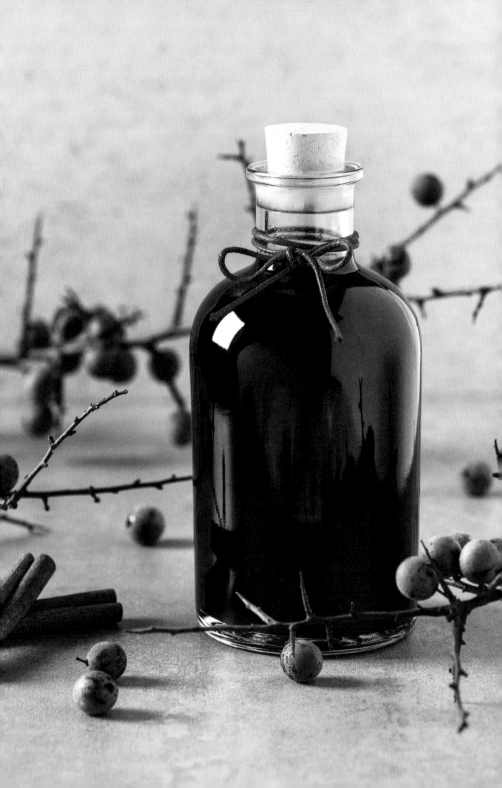

SLOE PORT

The sloes from your sloe gin (see page 132) still contain plenty of colour and flavour, with the added benefit that they are now soaked with gin. How wonderful that these gin-infused berries can be used twice in the making of a beautiful deep-red sloe port.

Makes approx. 1 litre

INGREDIENTS

The sloes that you have used to make your sloe gin

70 cl red wine (I like to use claret)

100 g caster sugar

200 ml brandy

METHOD

Put the sloes, wine and caster sugar into a 1-litre jar and shake to dissolve the sugar. Store in a cool, dark cupboard.

Leave for three weeks, giving it a little shake now and then when you remember.

After the three weeks, add the brandy, shake well and leave for at least three months before straining.

As with sloe gin, there's a fair bit of waiting around before you can sample your sloe port but, believe me, it's well worth it!

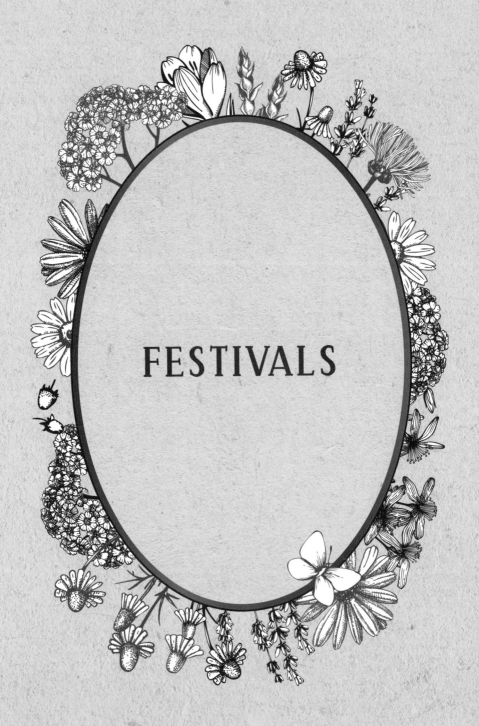

FESTIVALS

The lives of our Celtic forefathers were dominated by "the wheel of the year", which was made up of eight distinct festivals. These dictated to them when the season was right to sow, plough, harvest, celebrate and take some rest. The wheel turns continually according to the position of the sun, and represents the never-ending cycle of the birth, death and rebirth of nature. The seasons are still incredibly important as our very existence relies completely on abundant harvests. Even though we can now pretty much eat fruit and vegetables all year round, nothing tastes as delicious as food harvested in season that has been locally sourced or foraged.

MAY DAY

Other names for May Day: Beltane

This ancient Celtic celebration is known as Beltane, which is a Celtic word meaning "fires of Bel". It begins on 30 April and continues until 1 May. It is a festival to welcome the coming of summer, with anticipation of the abundant fertility of the year. Beltane rituals would often include courting; young couples would collect blossoms in the woods, make love and commit to marriages of a year and a day known as "handfastings". These handfasting ceremonies involved the tying together of hands with a red cord in a figure of eight for the duration of the ceremony. The hands would later be untied to symbolize that the union has been entered into with free will, and the couple would then "jump the broomstick" to denote moving from their old life to a new one.

Celts lit huge bonfires celebrating the return of light and fertility to the Earth. Single men and women would jump over the fire to attract a partner, and even pregnant women would jump through the fire to ensure a trouble-free birth.

The origins of the maypole hark back to ancient times when tree spirits were worshipped, and indeed the first maypoles were tall, slender trees, usually birch. These were felled and taken to the village where they had their branches taken off, leaving just a few at the top to be adorned with garlands and blossom. The finding, decorating and erecting of the village maypole was an important part of community life, becoming the focal point for dancing and merrymaking.

HARVEST

Other names for Harvest:
Harvest Festival, Lughnasadh, Lammas

Harvest is one of the oldest known festivals. It is traditionally celebrated in August on the harvest moon or on the full moon that is nearest to the autumn equinox. The word "Lammas" is derived from "Loaf Mass" in reference to the first grain being harvested, which would make the first loaf and begin the whole harvesting cycle. Lughnasadh, named after the pagan god Lugh, involved village gatherings with ritual ceremonies and much feasting.

It's the season when fruit is ripening, the grain is ready and we are thankful for the food on our tables.

The success or failure of the crop was a source of anxiety for our Celtic ancestors, and honouring gods and goddesses with a little inducement in the form of the first loaf was vital to ensure the success of the next year's harvest. In one Celtic story, a goddess, the Grain Mother, is heavily pregnant with a daughter, Persephone. Persephone signifies the fertile seed that will be placed into the earth; she will sleep all winter and emerge in the springtime, bringing new life with her. Persephone's father is the sun god, Lugh, who is sometimes called John Barleycorn or the Green Man; he embodies the spirit of the grain and will surrender his life to the harvest every Lammas when the first corn is cut.

After the medieval harvest had successfully been gathered in, the "gleaning bell" would be rung, signalling that the poorer women could make their way onto the fields to gather up any remaining useable crops.

HALLOWEEN

*Other names for Halloween: Samhain, All Souls' Night,
November Eve, Ancestor Night, All Hallow's Eve*

The tradition of Halloween, celebrated on 31 October, is often thought to have come from America, but it actually originated in Britain. It grew out of the ancient Celtic festival of Samhain, which was one of the major events of "The Wheel of the Year", marking the end of the light half of the year and the beginning of winter.

With the arrival of November came the faeries who would blast every growing plant with their freezing breath, ruining all that was left in the fields or hedgerows.

A tradition that began in the Middle Ages and lasted until around the eighteenth century was "souling", whereby children went from house to house singing rhymes and saying prayers for the dead in return for food. Each "soul cake" they received as payment for their songs meant that a soul was freed from purgatory and could ascend to heaven, and this was possibly the origin of trick or treating.

In 1891, the Reverend M. P. Holme of Cheshire wrote down this traditional souling song, told to him by a little girl from the local school:

"Soul, soul, a soul cake!
I pray thee, good missus, a soul cake!
One for Peter, two for Paul,
Three for Him what made us all!
Soul cake, soul cake, please good missus, a soul cake."

YULE

Other names for Yule: Winter Solstice, Christmas, Yuletide

A BRIEF HISTORY OF YULE

Yule is traditionally celebrated on the winter solstice, around 21 December, when darkness has reached its peak and daylight hours begin to lengthen. The Celts thought the sun stood still for twelve days over the Yule period; to conquer the darkness and protect themselves from evil spirits, they dragged a huge oak log into the house to burn. The log would be decorated with holly, pinecones and ivy, splashed with ale and then lit with a piece of the previous year's Yule log. Once burned, the log's ashes were valuable treasures said to have medicinal and magical powers that were able to guard against evil.

Until the fourth century, Yule was celebrated by pagans throughout Europe. Then Pope Julius I adopted 25 December as the date of the birth of Christ, and by the eleventh century the word "Christmas" had replaced "Yule" in most of England. By Tudor times, Christmas at court was celebrated by magnificent banquets, often with a "Lord of Misrule" who would caricature the court alongside an "Abbot of Unreason" who would ridicule the Church.

In the sixteenth and seventeenth centuries, Puritans put paid to Christmas celebrations as they believed them to be *"encouraging gluttony, drunkenness, sexual licence and public disorder"*, banning it altogether in 1647 along with Easter and Whitsun.

Christmas as we know it was pretty much a Victorian invention with the introduction of many familiar customs such as mince pies, holly, ivy, mistletoe and hospitality to our neighbours. Instead of burning the traditional Yule log as our Celtic ancestors did, we replaced this custom with the now familiar Yule log cake decorated to look like a tree branch.

WASSAIL

Other names for Wassailing: Apple Howling

Wassailing originated in Anglo-Saxon times, and is carried out to this day between Christmas Day and Twelfth Night. Wassailing is a ceremonial ritual that is believed to prepare apple trees for the coming year by awakening their spirit, thus ensuring they bear fruit. The spirit is believed to live in the oldest tree in the orchard and this particular tree is the centre of attention for the ceremony – in Somerset the spirit is known as "The Apple Tree Man".

A wassail king and queen lead the celebrations and are followed by the whole village, who are keen to join in with the noisy revelry. The wassailers process from orchard to orchard, making as much noise as possible: bashing pots and pans, shouting and singing, and more recently by firing shotguns, in order to scare away any wicked demons and awaken the sleeping tree spirit. Everyone gathers around the oldest tree and watches the wassail queen place a piece of alcohol-soaked bread into its branches. The wassail drink was traditionally a warm cider or ale with honey and spices, sometimes with the addition of an egg or two. This is passed around in a large bowl, with revellers shouting the traditional "wassail" greeting as it goes from person to person.

Any leftover cider is thrown at the tree and, just to make sure that the spirit is awake, more gunshots are fired into the branches. Wassailing wasn't just reserved for apple trees; plums and pears and any other fruit could be wassailed, too.

FINAL THOUGHTS

Interest in foraging is most definitely making a comeback as people become more concerned about the sustainability and origins of their food. Living through a pandemic made us look closer to home, searching out local suppliers and growers to fill our larders. Foraging is about as close to home as you can get as well as having the benefit of fresh air, exercise and proven improvements to our mental health – and it's free!

Foraging makes you more aware of the countryside around you. Even if you live in a city there are still lots of open spaces and parks for you to explore. You'll become guardians of the land and begin to notice any threat to our trees and hedgerows and hopefully do your best to help them flourish. Urban foragers will become experts in seeking out wild foods growing freely in the most surprising of places; all you need is bags of enthusiasm and enough curiosity to become more in tune with nature.

So, put on your walking boots, grab a basket, pop this guide in your pocket and get going on your exciting foraging adventure.

Good luck.

INDEX

Alexanders	28
Beech	46
Betony	82
Birch	48
Blackberry	81, 84, 124–125
Blackthorn	131, 132, 147
Borage	68
Burdock	86
Camomile	88
Chickweed	34
Chicory	90
Comfrey	50
Cow parsley	44
Crab apple	134
Daisy	52
Damsons	145
Dandelion	22, 24, 70–71, 72–73
Dog rose	54, 130
Elder	
Elder	45, 56
Ground elder	35
Elderberry	120–121

Fat hen 119

Garlic

    Crow garlic 35

    Garlic mustard 58

    Wild garlic 23, 32, 38–39

Gorse 69

Hawthorn 45, 60

Hazelnut 92, 122–123

Holly 136

Honeysuckle 80, 94

Horseradish 144

Horsetail 96

Juniper 98

Mallow 100

Meadowsweet 102

Mistletoe 138

Mugwort 104

Mullein 106

Nettle 23, 26, 36–37

Oak 140

Pignuts 69

Pine 131

Plantain 108

Poppy 62, 74–75

Primrose 64

Rowan 110

Sea buckthorn 116

Self-heal 81, 112

St John's Wort 114

Sweet chestnut 144

Violet 30

Walnuts 119

Wild cherry 118

Willow 142

Wild strawberry 118

Wild thyme 68

Wood sorrel 34

Yarrow 66

Image credits

Cover images: engraving illustrations © Yevheniia Lytvynovych/Shutterstock.com, butterfly © Yevheniia Lytvynovych/Shutterstock.com, background texture © Charunee Yodbun/Shutterstock.com, quarterbind texture © Art_Textures/Shutterstock.com
Insides: pp.4–5 © Cheplo Danil Vitalevich/Shutterstock.com; pp.6–7 © James Harrison/Shutterstock.com; pp.8–9 © Aleksey Mnogosmyslov/Shutterstock.com; pp.10–11, 14–15, 16–17, 22–23, 44–45, 80–81, 130–131 © Bodor Tivadar/Shutterstock.com; pp.12–13 © Lunov Mykola/Shutterstock.com; pp.18, 40, 76, 126, 148 © Yevheniia Lytvynovych/Shutterstock.com; pp.18–19, 20, 40–41, 42, 76–77, 78, 126–127, 128, 148–147, 156 © Charunee Yodbun/Shutterstock.com; pp.20, 42, 78, 128, 156 © Yevheniia Lytvynovych/Shutterstock.com; p.21 © Erkki Makkonen/Shutterstock.com; p.24 © kzww/Shutterstock.com; pp.24, 27, 29, 31, 33, 47, 49, 51, 53, 55, 57, 59, 61, 63, 65, 67, 83, 85, 87, 89, 91, 93, 95, 97, 99, 101, 103, 105, 107, 109, 111, 113, 115, 117, 133, 135, 137, 139, 141, 143 – background texture © Paladin12/Shutterstock.com; p.26 © nada54/Shutterstock.com; p.28 © PFMphotostock/Shutterstock.com; p.30 © alwih/Shutterstock.com; p.32 © 1928374166/Shutterstock.com; p.34 – chickweed © Morphart Creation/Shutterstock.com, wood sorrel © Morphart Creation/Shutterstock.com; p.35 – crow garlic © 772884181/Shutterstock.com, ground elder © FarbaKolerova/Shutterstock.com; p.36 © Konrad Mostert/Shutterstock.com; p.38 © Anna Shepulova/Shutterstock.com; p.43 © Torkiat8/Shutterstock.com; p.46 © Ihor Hvozdetskyi/Shutterstock.com; p.48 © Leonid Ikan/Shutterstock.com; p.50 © Anna Gratys/Shutterstock.com; p.52 © G-Arabul/Shutterstock.com; p.54 © Digoarpi/Shutterstock.com; p.56 © inimma/Shutterstock.com; p.58 © Nadya So/Shutterstock.com; p.60 © Maria Popa Photo/Shutterstock.com; p.62 © Serhii Brovko/Shutterstock.com; p.64 © bonilook/Shutterstock.com; p.66 © Sunbunny Studio/Shutterstock.com; p.67 – borage © Ja Raduga/Shutterstock.com, wild thyme © Hudozhnica_Ananas/Shutterstock.com; p.68 – gorse © Morphart Creation/Shutterstock.com, pignuts © Summersdale Publishers Ltd; p.70 © Christine Iverson; p.72 © Christine Iverson; p.74 © natalia bulatova/Shutterstock.com; p.79 © Ase/Shutterstock.com; p.82 © barmalini/Shutterstock.com; p.84 © ch_ch/Shutterstock.com; p.86 © Melanie Hobson/Shutterstock.com; p.88 © Thirteen/Shutterstock.com; p.90 © Andrey Venhlovskyi/Shutterstock.com; p.92 © Ian Grainger/Shutterstock.com; p.94 © krolya25/Shutterstock.com; p.96 © vaivirga/Shutterstock.com; p.98 © Melica/Shutterstock.com; p.100 © aniana/Shutterstock.com; p.102 © doroninanatalie4/Shutterstock.com; p.104 © wasanajai/Shutterstock.com; p.106 © Andriy Solovyov/Shutterstock.com; p.108 © Mr. Meijer/Shutterstock.com; p.110 © Anna Listarova/Shutterstock.com; p.112 © Svetlanko/Shutterstock.com; p.114 © Burkhard Trautsch/Shutterstock.com; p.116 © Petr Tkachev/Shutterstock.com; p.118 ¬– wild strawberry © Komleva/Shutterstock.com, wild cherry © NataLima/Shutterstock.com; p.119 – fat hen © Morphart Creation/Shutterstock.com, walnuts © DiViArt/Shutterstock.com; p.120 © Madeleine Steinbach/Shutterstock.com; p.122 © Justyna Pankowska/Shutterstock.com; p.124 © Anna_Pustynnikova/Shutterstock.com; p.129 © LilKar/Shutterstock.com; p.132 © Ihor Hvozdetskyi/Shutterstock.com; p.134 © kukuruxa/Shutterstock.com; p.136 © Kim Ferguson Photography/Shutterstock.com; p.138 © Hartmut Goldhahn/Shutterstock.com; p.140 © Editor77/Shutterstock.com; p.142 © Oleksandr Filatov/Shutterstock.com; p.144 – sweet chestnut © umiko/Shutterstock.com, horseradish © Morphart Creation/Shutterstock.com; p.145 © lamnee/Shutterstock.com; p.146 © Oksana_Schmidt/Shutterstock.com; p.155 © DUSAN ZIDAR/Shutterstock.com; p.160 © lola_art/Shutterstock.com

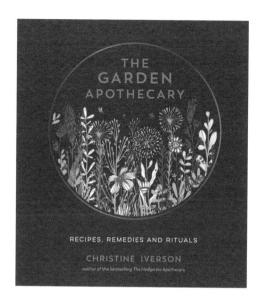

THE GARDEN APOTHECARY
Recipes, Remedies and Rituals

Hardback

ISBN: 978-1-78783-979-3

£14.99

Learn how to make the most of your common garden plants like the herbalists of the past

Unlock the sustainable and ethical art of the apothecarist, and explore its rich folklore and history. Discover the hidden delights in your own garden and how to use them to make delicious edible treats, herbal cures and restorative beauty products. With photographs to help you safely identify edible plants and tips on how best to prepare and preserve your finds, this is the essential guide to enjoying the home-grown riches of your garden.

"Christine Iverson has translated her love for nature and her skills for foraging into this practical guide."

THE TIMES

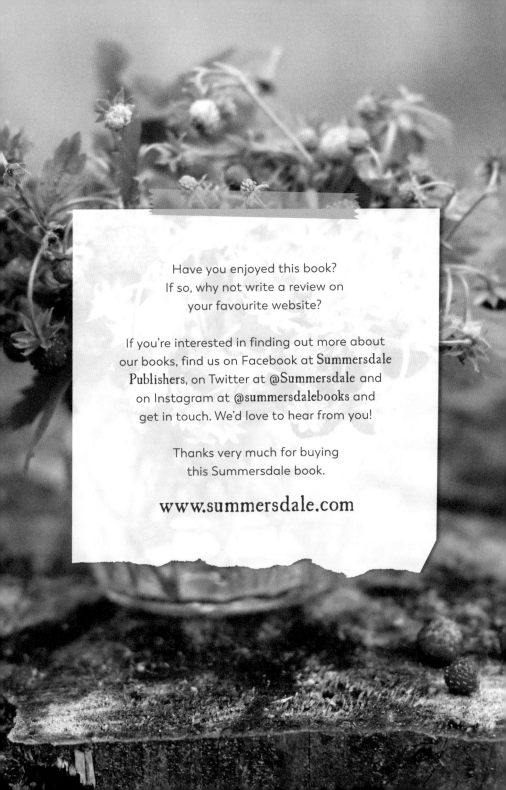

Have you enjoyed this book?
If so, why not write a review on
your favourite website?

If you're interested in finding out more about
our books, find us on Facebook at Summersdale
Publishers, on Twitter at @Summersdale and
on Instagram at @summersdalebooks and
get in touch. We'd love to hear from you!

Thanks very much for buying
this Summersdale book.

www.summersdale.com